Personality Strength and Psychochemical Energy

By the same author:

Nutrition and Your Mind

Personality Strength and Psychochemical Energy

How to Increase Your Total Performance

by

George Watson

Harper & Row, Publishers

New York, Hagerstown, San Francisco, London

To Marilyn

FIRST EDITION

Designer: Janice Stern

Library of Congress Cataloging in Publication Data

Watson, George, 1912–
                    Personality strength and psychochemical energy.

  Includes Index.
  1. Personality. 2. Performance. 3. Nutrition—
Psychological Aspects. 4. Odors—Testing. I. Title.
BF698.W383   613.2   79–1690
ISBN 0-06-014587-0

---

79 80 81 82 83 10 9 8 7 6 5 4 3 2 1

Contents

Acknowledgments

I am indebted to many who have worked with me, but I am unable to name them here. The reason for this is the unfortunate—and totally unexpected—volume of mail (many tens of thousands) and telephone calls generated by my book *Nutrition and Your Mind*. Universities and scientists I named in the book were burdened with constant appeals for my address and telephone number, and with appeals for references to physicians. The book was published in 1972 (Harper & Row); since that time the climate has changed radically, and it is no longer difficult to find a physician interested in pursuing individual psychochemistry.

I must, however, acknowledge my very great debt to W. D. Currier, M.D. Over a twenty-year period he has given freely of his time, provided facilities when I needed them, and provided the services of his staff of excellent nurses. Of these I owe a particular debt of gratitude to his chief nurse, Mrs. Clem Frindt, who helped me in so many ways. The kinds of assistance given to this research endeavor by Dr. Currier and his staff are beyond purchase, and my gratitude is profound.

I am particularly grateful to my editor at Harper & Row, Frances McCullough, whose intelligent and judicious editing has improved this book immensely.

GEORGE WATSON

1

A Strong Personality

One quiet Sunday morning I was writing in my study when I heard what was definitely a shot. It was fired from either a large-caliber revolver or a hunting rifle—and apparently not too far away from where I was sitting.

I stepped quickly out the sliding glass door, looked around— expecting to see someone with a gun hunting the wild deer that roamed in the north meadow.

I saw no one. The shot must have come from farther away than it had sounded. Our neighbor lived about a quarter of a mile across the meadow and was something of a gun collector. I guessed he must have fired one of them.

That afternoon I found out that he had indeed pulled a trigger. The gun was pointed in his direction. The shot was deflected when his wife hit his arm.

We had been invited by the Canfields,* our only neighbors, to come over that afternoon for a social hour or two. When we arrived, Ruby Canfield said, "I'm so glad you've come. Roy is upset, and there's been an accident."

---

* All the names used in this book have been arbitrarily assigned to protect the identities of the real persons involved.

Roy Canfield was thirty-eight, headed his own construction company, had two sons, twelve and fourteen. He and Ruby had been married sixteen years or so, and I had known them most of that time.

Ruby said, "Roy almost shot himself. He's in the study."

I went in and found him sitting by the fireplace reading the *National Geographic*. There was a small bandage on his chin, and he looked a little pale.

"Ruby told me you had some kind of accident. What happened?"

He said he really didn't know what had happened. He remembered cleaning a revolver and "playing around with it." He also remembered the shot. Pointing to the bandage on his chin, he said, "Powder burn."

Neither he nor his wife seemed overly concerned. This puzzled me, for *I* was concerned. Was this an attempted suicide? I could hardly believe so. Roy Canfield was to me the least likely person to consider such a thing. He was a big, muscular fellow—over six feet tall at about two hundred pounds. Young and confident, the outdoor type: kept horses, rode almost daily, hunted, fished, and all the rest. I had always believed that he was easily the strongest person I had ever known—physically, mentally, and emotionally.

I asked him if he was upset or depressed about anything, and he said, "Nothing unusual." But he also said that his "thinking" had been off for a few weeks or so. "I just can't seem to get my head clear."

"How do you feel right now?" I asked.

"Sort of dazed."

I went out to my car and got my bag. We had driven the short distance across the meadow since the creek was running high from late spring rains.

Mine is not a physician's bag, but a researcher's. It contains a variety of nutritional biochemicals, including my Psychochemical Odor Test kit. This test provides a quick and reliable index of the way a person is breaking down food to create energy in the brain and nervous system.

The Canfields knew about my work and about the test. I'd been working on its development for many years, and once in a while I would test Roy just to confirm my clinical opinion that he was not only "normal" biochemically, but also very stable. His scores were virtually all the same, and unless he had the flu or something, always "normal."

Today, however, his psychochemical profile was way off. He was not turning blood sugar into energy fast enough to meet the needs of his brain and other body tissues. In fact, his oxidation rate was as slow as those of some of our seriously ill research patients. No wonder he felt "dazed" and couldn't remember what had happened when the gun went off. He simply hadn't known what he was doing.

Since it is not under conscious control, this kind of behavior is "psychochemical." The brain is not functioning normally. Consequently such behavior is unplanned, has no meaning or motive, and thus falls outside of the area of psychological understanding and explanation.

Ruby came into the study and asked me what I thought. I said the shot looked like one of those things—a psychochemical response—since Roy's mental processes were so far from normal.

"I figured it must have been something like that, abnormal or whatever," Ruby said. I reassured her that in my mind there was little doubt but that the shot was unintentional. She said she just wished they didn't have all those guns lying around. "Anything might happen."

I told Roy to drink a large glass of orange juice and gave him a triple dose of the vitamin-mineral formula (see page 64) we use for slow oxidizers. The nutrients in this formula are designed to speed up brain processes. I decided to stay right there with him until his biochemical balance shifted back to normal. I checked him on the odor test every half hour, repeating the vitamin-mineral-orange-juice combination each time. Two hours later his scores on the Psychochemical Odor Test were about normal, and Roy said, "I'm okay. I'm out of it."

Before I left I suggested he try to see his physician the next day for a physical examination and routine blood tests. We had to find out what had caused the shift in his metabolism, and the first place to look would be at his general physical condition.

Roy called me several days later and told me his doctor said he could find nothing wrong. "In fact," Roy said, "the doctor told me I appeared to be in great shape, and whatever I was doing to keep this way, I should just keep on doing it." Then Roy asked me if I was free and could he come over and talk to me about something personal.

Here is a brief summary of what he told me:

About ten months before his construction firm had decided to bid on a large government project—one involving something around twenty million dollars—and they had to meet a deadline in an unusually short time since their decision to try for the contract was made so late.

This meant long hours at work, little sleep, and meals consisting largely of luncheon meats (cold cuts), cheese, nuts, potato chips, and "gallons" of coffee, brought in by secretaries and consumed over a calculator.

Roy said that after they had successfully met the deadline he went home, took a week off, and slept for twelve hours a night for a week. "But," he said, "I've never felt good since. At times I'm afraid—almost panicky—that our bid was so low that if it is accepted I'll lose maybe a million or so." He added that he was seriously considering getting out of the construction business because the pressure was beginning to get to him. "Deals like this never used to bother me. And I've lost money before, but I always figured to make it up on the next job. I guess I'm losing my nerve. I don't have that old confidence anymore."

This story all added up to one thing to me. While words such as "confidence" and "nerve" signify mental and emotional states when one uses psychological language, in my view, however, whether one is "confident" and has "nerve" ultimately depends upon the amount of energy one is creating and using in his nervous system.

Since Roy said he was losing his confidence and his nerve, I translated this into my language—nutritional biochemistry—to mean that somehow he had lost his former ability to produce the very high levels of physical and mental strength that had powered his strong personality and carried him to his unusual business success.

Where, one must ask, does one begin to try to find out what had happened to Canfield, since the human body is an almost incredible complex of interacting biochemical systems? His physician had checked most of the obvious possibilities, such as heart, lungs, kidneys, liver, and thyroid function, and since these were all "normal," he pronounced Roy to be in good health. And, in terms of just these tests, he was.

But—and this is a very large "but"—in addition to the factors Canfield's doctor checked, there remains a "gray area" in medical knowledge outside the range of interest and training of even the best physicians, and that concerns the way the tissues of the body convert food into energy and what possible tests could be used to assess these processes.

Consequently, Canfield's physician said the problem was simply one of "nerves," and suggested he take five milligrams of a mild tranquilizer twice a day.

After Canfield told me this, I sent him to our lab for the group of blood tests that we had found to be useful indicators of the way one's tissues are creating energy.

As I suspected, we found him to be what we call a "slow oxidizer," one of four psychochemical types. The others are "fast oxidizers," "variable oxidizers," and "suboxidizers." These will be discussed in detail in a later chapter. For the present let me just say that these are abnormal patterns of metabolism—of creating energy. And all four types have one thing in common: a functional disturbance in the manner in which body cells turn food into energy, while the phrase "functional disturbance" indicates that these abnormal patterns are correctable.

Since the brain and the nervous system use proportionately more energy than any other of the body's organs, when there is a misfunction in the energy cycles, the first adverse effects are found in one's thinking, feeling, and behavior.

In Roy Canfield's case, something had interfered with his ability to convert blood sugar and other nutrients into energy. The psychological result was loss of nerve, loss of confidence, and recurring attacks of anxiety.

As I said earlier, Canfield was one of the strongest persons— mentally, physically, and emotionally—that I had ever known. But this was true only as long as his biochemical functioning was at its peak. His "strong personality" vanished when the cells in his nervous system cut off the power.

One thinks of two questions at this point: what caused the power failure? and can the biochemical systems which failed be restored to their previous high level of energy production?

The answer to the first of these questions is fairly easy in this particular case. Canfield was not ill and had, before his slump began, been going full blast. But he was nearing the age of forty, and there is such a thing as biochemical erosion: people can and do wear themselves down—some much more rapidly than others. It has been my experience that really strong people such as Roy Canfield simply do not know what it means to "take it easy," since they never really experience the *feeling* of simply being exhausted. They don't *appear* to need much sleep, *apparently* can skip meals without ill effect, while working seventy or eighty hours a week, right up to the time they begin to fall apart.

By the phrases "biochemical erosion" and "wear themselves down" I don't mean the inevitable degenerative changes that occur in all of us, which are generally referred to as "aging." What I am referring to is the depletion, the "using up," of replaceable *nutrients* which are crucial to the cells' functioning. The most important of these substances are minute quantities of trace elements (minerals such as selenium, chromium, etc.) and vitamins which are parts of enzymes (complexes of proteins and vitamins), and minerals such as calcium, potassium, sodium, and iron.

Enzymes literally turn food into energy, repair tissues, and make hormones. The repair and replacement of enzymes goes on constantly, and of course cannot be accomplished if the needed materials are not available from the food one eats. If one does not regularly replace what has been used up, one is on the downslide biochemically. This is biochemical erosion, and this is what caused Roy Canfield's power failure: he was using his energy-producing capacities faster than he was making repairs with replacements.

The second question was whether biochemical systems that fail owing to overwork and inadequate maintenance can be restored to their former efficiency.

The answer is "yes," with qualifications: the general health of the individual (such as absence of high blood pressure, diabetes, and other kinds of organic illness) makes a difference. So does his "regenerative age"—the index of how long his negative nutritional balance has been in existence. Persons with long histories of nutritional neglect, particularly if such neglect occurred in childhood or adolescence, have limited abilities for self-repair.

Those with what we may call long regenerative ages may be helped, but the extent of recovery is not complete, and the time required to accomplish such recovery may be as long as two or three years.

In terms of the conditions just summarized, in medical language one would say the "prognosis" for Roy Canfield's full recovery was excellent. He was in very good physical condition by ordinary medical standards, and his regenerative age was apparently quite short. With Roy Canfield we could expect good recovery within two to four months.

These were rough estimations. But they are based on about thirty years of clinical observation and research, and are useful in judging one's own condition and projecting one's own expectations. If you're twenty years old and have been living on junk food for about the last six, don't expect any miracles when you adopt a rational diet. Improvement will show almost at once, but the steady process of full recovery is gradual.

There is "full" recovery, and there is "partial" recovery. But to me the most exciting phenomenon is the possibility of *increasing* an individual's personality strength and higher achievement potential. Not only can one recover from the kind of biochemical slide experienced by Roy Canfield. It is frequently possible for individuals to come out of it functioning at higher levels of aspiration and achievement than they had known previously at their very best.

Since Canfield had been an enormously strong person by anyone's standards before his intensive lifestyle caught up with bio-chemical reality, my highest hope was to try to get him back to where he had been before. He said he wanted to "get out of the construction business." I wanted him to stay with and continue his success.

Canfield Construction had started modestly about twenty years before building single-family homes. They then added apartments, then bid on public buildings, built city and county roads, and then began to bid on sections of state expressways. At the time Roy began to show signs of running down, they were working on big projects halfway across the country.

For all Canfield's drive, courage, and business acumen, almost unbelievably he still possessed one of those untapped reservoirs of great strength and higher aspirations that frequently manifest themselves when the right person receives *all* of the nutritional biochemicals he is genetically capable of using. I call this indi-vidually tailored, intensive treatment *orthonutrition*, which means, ideally, supplying all of the correct foods, plus nutritional supplements, that a person can utilize. And, since one's nutrition-al requirements vary, owing to a variety of reasons (illness, weather, etc.), the orthonutritional program provides a simple and reliable test one can use to adjust one's food and vitamin-mineral intake as needed. This is what I call the Psychochemical Odor Test. For example, if you don't feel as good as you think you should, the Psychochemical Odor Test can tell you whether the problem is a nutritional one, and if so, what to do about it. Knowing oneself psychochemically is the key to maximum psy-chological, physical, and emotional strength. Very few people ever achieve this goal through casual eating.

After Canfield started on his orthonutritional program he was back at work—full speed—apparently functioning in the man-ner that had made him so successful.

My contacts with him became infrequent, since he was often

away from home, checking his varied projects. I really had no firm idea of how well he was doing. On occasion, we would meet at a social event, and I would ask him how he was and how his business was getting along, and he'd say he never felt better and that everything was going great—which I interpreted as a mere social platitude.

But about two years later I turned to the financial pages of the Sunday paper. The heading of one column at once caught my attention: "Canfield Construction Wins Bid to Build Oil Docking Facilities in Near East."

In this chapter I have mentioned four psychochemical types: the fast oxidizer, the slow oxidizer, the variable oxidizer, and the suboxidizer. I have also indicated that these are abnormal biochemical conditions, resulting in lowered psychological functioning. In addition to the "normal" person, however, my experience with people such as Roy Canfield suggests that there exists an untold number of supernormal people with undetected capabilities. These people grope their way through life, having no inkling of their unrecognized and thus unrealized potential.

2

Food, Mood, and the Sense
of Smell

He held a prescription vial half-filled with wafershaped pills, and while he was talking he would toss the vial sharply from his right to his left hand and back again—as a pitcher does a baseball.

This irritating and distracting motion magnified the edgy unpleasantness of what this thirty-eight-year-old man was saying—and had been saying for what now seemed to have been a very long time.

"If you really knew her, could see and hear her in action, morning, noon, midnight, any time at all"—the words tumbled and rushed over each other—"well, you'd begin to see *my* side of this thing. Really, my reaction to my wife has little to do with *me*. I just happen to be the accidental victim."

I interrupted, having heard far more than enough of his self-justification. He had walked out on his wife and family.

"What's in the vial?" I asked, steering the talk to a new track.

"Penicillin," he said. "Really great for strep throat." In a quick motion he tossed the vial toward me and, surprisingly, I caught it. I took the cap off and sniffed the contents. To me they had a faint minty odor. I replaced the cap and tossed the vial back.

"Have you ever smelled penicillin wafers?" I asked. I was hoping to lead him into an informal odor response test.

With a quick motion he opened the vial, placed it under his nose, and drew back sharply, exclaiming, "Wow! That's some powerful gas!"

A devious ruse on my part, particularly in a social setting. But I was determined to discover a strategy which would enable me to get an insight into the biochemistry of the young man sitting across the coffee table from me.

I'd known "Paul Carter" socially for some time. He taught engineering physics at a nearby university. He also was a technical consultant to the government, and was said to have played a significant role in some of the spectacular successes of the space program.

One of our general research aims was to gather information on as wide a sample of temperaments as possible, and Professor Carter's reputation for unpredictability certainly qualified him as research material in our view. I had been told that he was "brilliant beyond the reach of intelligence tests, but as erratic and explosive emotionally as he was brilliant and creative mentally."

I was further informed: "There are days when he arrives at the laboratory really wild and sort of crazy, with a certain look in his eye that scares you. Yet there are other times—fortunately more frequent—when he is as soft and gentle as a church librarian. Consequently, many of his subordinates hate him—those who've been roughed up on his bad days—and these appear to be getting more frequent. If so, I'm afraid we'll have to let him go or lose many highly valuable members of his staff. Two have resigned this last month. What we are looking for is someone who can help him. Several of your former patients suggested that we try to get you."

Here, obviously, was a prime chance to enlarge our understanding of some of the relationships between temperament and body chemistry.

Although the penicillin wafers that Professor Carter had just smelled might appear to be unusual material to use for an odor test, they were not too different from certain of our standard laboratory sniff test materials. In our search for sensitive odor indicators we had screened hundreds of drugs, foods, cosmetics—just about everything you could think of. I personally had come across penicillin wafers as a test source when my physician gave them to me for a throat infection. Subsequently, I had been able to correlate shifts in odor test responses to them that matched our standard test materials.

The reason Carter had such a strong reaction to the penicillin wafers was that his body chemistry was off: he was breaking down blood sugar in his tissues at a very rapid rate. My own mild reaction to the wafers was normal. This problem will be discussed in detail in Chapter 3. But for the present the following paragraphs should be sufficient.

What a given substance smells like depends a good deal upon the general biochemical state of the person doing the smelling. If I can manipulate your biochemical condition, say, stimulate your nervous system to burn sugar more rapidly, I can also thereby alter your sense of smell.

Individuals vary widely in the fluctuations of their odor responses, just as they vary widely in biochemical stability. In general, the more stable a person is psychologically, the more unvarying and "normal" are the biochemical processes occurring in his or her body tissues. Conversely, the less stable a person is mentally and emotionally, the more variable in both rate and kind are the biochemical reactions taking place within him. Your sense of smell reflects the chemistry of your body. In a word, if you will let me screen you on the Psychochemical Odor Test, you will also be letting me get a glimpse into your psychological state.

Such a glimpse is exactly what I had just had when Paul Carter described the penicillin wafers as smelling like "some powerful gas." I related his particular response to penicillin with the biochemical pattern of the most common psychochemical type—the *fast* oxidizer. And I might add that Paul Carter was a very fast oxidizer indeed.

One of the characteristics one observes in people perhaps too frequently—particularly in men—is the refusal even to admit the possibility that there could be something about them that needs attention and correction. This fault is bad enough when it shows up, say, as a refusal to see a dentist for a routine checkup. But when the point in question involves what some like to think of as the "mind" or "personality," the block against admitting a correctable defect is generally insurmountable.

In the many social conversations I had with Dr. Carter one symptom of this kind of ego resistance had soon shown itself. The main thrust of his social comments seemed to be heavily laced with remarks pointing out the weakness, stupidities, and general shortcomings of others, including his wife. At times his outspoken, blunt criticism of others was quite embarrassing.

When I was given background briefing on Carter, the first thing I was warned about was that, although he obviously needed help of some kind, my main objective should be to get him to seek and accept it.

Since I had found it difficult enough to help those who earnestly solicited help from me, I hardly found it to my taste to try to arrange a biochemical realignment in a patient *without* his knowledge, consent, or cooperation.

However, I had two small points of attack to try on Carter: his scientific curiosity and his occasional but intractable headaches. So, when he reacted strongly to his sniff test on the penicillin wafers, I appeared quite surprised—and I really was.

"They don't smell a bit like that to me, at all," I said emphatically.

I went on to explain what I thought accounted for our different reactions, and further commented that perhaps it would be a small matter to change his sense of smell so that his odor responses agreed with mine.

He positively bristled at this. "You really don't know anything about physics at all, do you?" He then carefully explained that penicillin had a specific molecular structure, and that particles from the wafers in the vial entered the nose, and that the shape of the molecules sort of "fit" into a corresponding shape of the sensory receptors at the back of the mouth and in the nose. The nerves, he said, carried this information about the molecular fit to the brain, where it was registered as a "certain smell."

This to me was a familiar and very limited type of hypothesis about olfactory reaction. I ignored it. Instead I said, "Perhaps the reason why your sense of smell is so far from normal is you're coming down with a cold—or even more likely that you've got a bad headache."

At this he seemed to relax a bit. "A good shot, but probably a lucky one. I do have the headache, and I only hope your guess about the cold is wrong."

I won this first real skirmish, for he agreed to borrow a small, six-sample odor kit from me and record his reactions under varying conditions of fatigue, emotional attitude (mood), and presence or absence of headache.

Lending him the odor test kit was the first move, I hoped, toward getting Professor Carter to become a full volunteer research subject. The goal was to have him agree to medical, psychological, and biochemical tests, together with whatever remedial measures might be appropriate.

Some time ago a physician friend from college days told me something one could only expect to learn from a person of long acquaintance. I was describing to him some of the bizarre and difficult psychological types—such as Paul Carter—that turn up in the offices of researchers.

"I couldn't stand it," he commented. "Whenever I get a troublesome, oddball patient, I simply refer him or her to another physician."

I guess my surprise at this disclosure somehow leaked into my facial expression. My colleague added, somewhat defensively, "I can't let anyone give me a bad time and undermine my self-confidence. I owe this to myself, to my family, and to the patients I *can* help, and who depend upon me."

But in research it is that difficult patient who forces one to think. The greater the trouble, the more likelihood of new insights. And it was trouble all the way with Paul Carter.

Barely two days after I had given him the odor kit I received a call from him telling me flatly that I must have made a frightful error, since the test odors almost never smelled the same on repeated testings!

His irritation at this discovery almost equaled my surprise. For the kit contained samples of six common materials that we had used in odor testing for many years, and on which we had recorded thousands of reports. And for psychochemically "normal" people, that is to say either established psychochemical types or normal test subjects, the different contexts of odor responses were almost always unvarying. Something was very much wrong with what Dr. Carter was telling me, and I needed to know just what that was. So I asked him to bring the kit and come to my lab for an extensive olfactory screening involving over two dozen test samples.

It was a rather different Paul Carter who arrived at my office on Saturday at just a half minute before the appointed hour of eleven. He said he hoped he "wasn't too early," adding that "when one works on planning space shots, there develops a tendency to carry precision timing over into everything else—appropriate or not." His manner was relaxed, and he had a tendency to smile.

After I'd run the complete series of odor tests on him, finding that his responses were surprisingly all about "normal," I asked him whether by any chance he had retested the odor of the penicillin wafers.

"I had to have the prescription refilled and the new wafers didn't smell anything at all like the old ones," he said.

"Did the new ones smell rather faint, and something like acetone—like nail polish remover?" I asked.

"How could you ever guess *that*," he said, "unless you spend a lot of time going around smelling different batches of penicillin wafers!"

Well, of course I *had* guessed, even though the guess wasn't exactly based upon chance. Odor descriptions of penicillin wafers as "acetone," "polish remover," or "some kind of solvent" are characteristic replies given by persons whose oxidation rate is a little slow, but almost normal. They are not burning blood sugar rapidly enough in the nervous system. And that distorts their perceptions.

My brief glimpses into Paul Carter's metabolic machinery were really beginning to spell chaos. I now had received hints of biochemical reactions from one extreme to the other, with a pause for normality. And I was beginning to get an idea of what was behind his complaint about something being wrong with the odor test kit I had given him. For there could be no other explanation for his report that "not one of the test odors in the kit hardly ever smelled the same on repeated testings" but that the person doing the smelling was incredibly unstable biochemically. That person was the volatile Professor Carter.

I was thus gradually becoming aware of the fact that I was in a rather difficult situation. To confirm my idea about Carter's variability would require real information—studies performed on blood samples taken under as wide a sampling of psychological conditions as Carter normally experienced. This would particularly require him to be tested when he felt, as my sources noted, "wild and sort of crazy, with a certain look in his eye that scares you."

The very thought of getting cooperation from him under such conditions almost stopped me. The whole prospect seemed beyond reality. I could never lure him to the clinical laboratory for tests at the appropriate times by ruses of any kind. He would have to know what his condition was, and also know that I was fully aware of the likelihood that he had extreme personal psychological difficulties.

It began to look as though the only chance there was of getting the information I needed was to level with him. But, because I had been warned about his resistance to psychological help, I hated to risk it. So I decided to fall back on the old rule of when in doubt do nothing. I would simply coach him on the use of the odor kit. After all, Carter was bright, and he just might, with a few hints, find out for himself some correlations between food, mood, and the sense of smell.

I therefore asked him if he would keep a record of what he ate, and also record his odor responses before breakfast, after lunch (about an hour), and at bedtime. I reassured him that there was nothing wrong with the kit I had given him, but explained that it had to be used systematically in order to reflect repeated patterns of responses to certain dietary habits. I also gave him a chart which outlined the principal patterns of odor responses for slow, normal, and fast oxidizers, explaining that some of the apparent confusion of shifting odors he had experienced could be understood if he were to try to fit his self-observations into these patterns. I also again emphasized the importance of recording odor responses at the times of headaches—reinforcing the idea that it was not unlikely we might uncover a clue that could lead to help.

I didn't hear from Professor Carter for almost a month. Then he called late one night and said he had time to come over and discuss the records he had been keeping.

It was again a pleasant, relaxed Carter who arrived right on time the following morning. I began to suspect that I'd only see him when he was pleasant—when he felt relaxed and normal enough to make and keep an appointment.

I glanced through the sheaf of notes he handed me and at once was struck by the number of recorded odor descriptions correlated with an unusually fast oxidation rate. Very often he had noted that he could detect no odors at all, only a penetrating "gassy" sensation in his nose and throat. This type of response is correlated with an extremely rapid breakdown in the tissues of sugar and other nutrients.

Almost unthinkingly I reacted with surprise. "Gosh, with responses like some of these I'm surprised you didn't feel something!"

He reacted instantly. "What do you mean 'feel something'?"

"Well," I replied, now a little cautiously, "in most cases, when a person's oxygen consumption is way up, perhaps they're anxious, tense, or excited. And once in a while they might even feel a little wild—like they're going to do something they don't want to do, say, smash something or even hit someone."

"Don't you mean, rather," he asked—and his voice now sounded strained—"that a tense, anxious, or excited person consumes more oxygen than a calm one? But you said just the reverse."

I agreed that if the fire bell rang in the night, the resulting fear would increase one's oxygen consumption. But I also said it was equally true that if for any *biochemical* reason one's oxidation rate was accelerated one's feelings would also be altered. I added that the biochemical reasons could be—and very often were—unsuspected nutritional ones.

This answer didn't satisfy Carter, and he came right back and asked how I could tell from merely reading the odor descriptions what the precipitating conditions might have been.

Of course he was right: I couldn't. But I had a legitimate out, for I had asked him to record both odor responses *and* mood. If he'd had an argument and was angry, for example, he *should* have noted it. But he had made no notations on this important subject. My unspoken belief was that he didn't record his hostile feelings because he didn't want to tip his hand—a very common reaction among emotionally disturbed people. However, it was my job to make him do just that, or we'd never get anywhere. But, in order to achieve this, I was first going to have to convince him that there was nothing wrong with his "mind."

I believed it most likely that at the heart of Carter's wish to hide or try to ignore his marked and perhaps even wild fluctuations in mood was that he had no idea at all what was causing them, and probably had no hope or thought that there was anything he could do about them. Like many of those whose ideas reflect the current establishment notions in psychology, he probably felt that his mind was some kind of mysterious psychic thing that simply possessed certain characteristics, and that for him these unfortunately included unusually wide variations in mood, feeling, and emotion.

My task was to try to get him to look at himself in a new context—a different frame of reference—where fuzzy words such as "mind," "personality," and "temperament" would lose their function to mask ignorance.

I have said it had been our experience that most of the progress we had made in gaining new insights into some of the basic psychochemical factors in behavior had been through the vexed business of trying to cope with the problems of really difficult people. But the likelihood hardly occurred to me at the time I began working with Paul Carter that his name would one day come to be linked in my mind with the identification of a new psychochemical type—the variable oxidizer.

There is an important concept in biochemistry called "homeostasis." This refers to the normal tendency of the body's processes to remain constant or stable under varying conditions. To cite one common example, the body has a rather elaborate system for keeping the sugar in the blood at an optimum functional level, even though there is a constant drain on one's reserves by the tissues to make energy.

In the language of homeostasis, a "psychochemical type" is a kind of malfunctioning or disturbance in the energy-producing and -regulating systems of the body. Such disturbances in homeostasis have profound effects upon thinking, feeling, and behavior, known as "homeoinstasis." The "in" in this word is negative, signifying absence of the normal constancy of functioning in the energy-producing and -control body systems.

In looking over the notes in which Dr. Carter recorded his reactions to the odor test, I was struck not only with the frequency of correlation of mood ("felt a little 'high' ") with a highly accelerated breakdown of blood sugar. I also noted, intermingled with a sprinkling of normal responses, a number of reactions at the extreme other end of the scale. These were indications of a very slow rate of glucose utilization, and the effect of this could only be most unfavorable. Moodiness, depression, anxiety, paranoia, aggressiveness, as well as other, more serious types of disorders, are the kinds of things associated with a grossly reduced rate of blood sugar and oxygen consumption in the brain and nervous system.

But perhaps most surprising in Carter's records was the fact that he had often recorded extreme shifts from fast to normal to very slow oxidation rates within a matter of a few hours. In all of my experience I had never come across such radical variability in homeostasis. I was here getting a glimpse of what perhaps lay behind Carter's "unpredictable temperament." But I needed more than a glimpse: Carter was a very rare bird who had to be studied very carefully.

After slowly going over all of his notations carefully, I finally told him that the most likely explanation for the variability of his odor responses was a direct relationship with a similar variability in the breakdown of nutritional biochemicals in his tissues, resulting in wide changes in mood, feeling, and even the kind of person one perceives oneself to be.

"Since you are a scientist," I said, "you no doubt would like to see this claim documented—like to see some correlated biochemical test data."

Carter smiled at this and nodded his head rather vigorously in agreement.

I then proposed a little experiment: for three days he would go on a high-purine protein diet, with a moderate fat intake but with a quite limited use of carbohydrates—almost no bread, fruit, sweets of any kind, etc.—together with certain non-starchy vegetables that I would suggest.

On the fourth morning he would allow us to perform some blood studies, among them a four-hour glucose tolerance test. He would continue to record his odor responses during this trial diet period, together with notations of his general psychological state—whether depressed, irritable, anxious, hostile, or whatever. I gave him a list of suggested meals for this three-day test period, emphasizing that it was essential to follow the prescribed diet.

In selecting the test diet for Carter—very much like the one recommended for fast oxidizers—I was guided by the preponderance of odor responses on his lists that indicated an unusually fast breakdown of blood sugar.

When he first gave me his lists of odor responses with the records of what he had eaten, I had noted that his food choices followed no easily discernible pattern. For example, one morning he would eat an orange, two or three dried figs, and a few walnuts, while the next day he would eat sausages and eggs. Since my own interests led me to think of foods in terms of their metabolic functions, I would have had to conclude from merely inspecting Carter's food lists that he must be very stable and could eat anything anytime without adverse effect. That is, until I also saw his records of odor responses. With these two types of information, however, it was an easy bet that the result of the wide variations in nutritional input was going to be reflected in his psychological stability.

After a brief discussion of the types of foods I wanted him to eat—and he said he liked all of them—he agreed to see for himself whether indeed his odor responses were linked to his diet and blood chemistry, and even to the way he felt and functioned.°

I suspected that Carter's fast breakdown of sugar was also correlated with his headaches, which he had failed to note on his

---

° Diets, dietary supplements, and sample menus are given in Chapter 7 for fast, slow, and suboxidizers.

lists. When I remarked this omission to him he said, "What's the use? I almost always have some kind of a headache." He had been through "all the best" medical clinics, he said, and no one had ever found anything physically wrong. Their answer was always the same: "See a psychiatrist," which he would not do, for reasons he did not disclose and I dared not inquire about.

In retrospect this seemingly sensible program just about terminated my relationship not only with Professor Carter, but with his colleagues who had recommended me to him.

The traumatic difficulties that were the outcome of my suggested "little experiment" with Carter would never have occurred had it not been for Carter's own disinclination to follow simple directions.

Because the fast oxidizer diet that I had given him is designed to retard the rapid breakdown of blood sugar, such a program can and does lead to unwanted psychological consequences when it is followed inappropriately—when, for example, sugar utilization is already too slow and the diet slows it down even further.

The arrangement was for Carter to go on the diet for three days, and then come in on the morning of the fourth day for his blood tests. When he failed to appear for the tests I assumed his schedule interfered, and that he would call me for another appointment—as he had done before.

I learned from a mutual colleague, however, that the initial effect of the diet was dramatic. Carter had had two days of feeling unusually good—high energy with little or no headache. On the basis of this limited experience he decided to stay on the diet for an indefinite period to "maximize the benefits."

Our colleague—a former patient of mine—also told me that he definitely noticed that Carter soon began to "sort of withdraw." Bursts of irritability would be followed by long periods of silence—very untypical behavior for him.

One really odd outcome of this whole episode was that Carter blamed *me* for making him "depressed almost to the point of self-destruction."

When I heard this I decided to forget about Carter for the present. I hoped that, perhaps given the opportunity to reflect, he might arrive at a different estimate of what had happened to him. In fact, in the press and urgency of dealing with other research patients I virtually forgot the whole Carter episode.

It must have been six months later at a meeting attended by several research scientists that I was approached by one of Carter's associates, who complimented me on what a "great job" I had done in "settling down" Carter!

This really surprised me, and I quickly declined the compliment.

"But," he protested, "Carter himself told me how much you had helped him."

Well, perhaps. I *had* given him the odor kit with detailed instructions on its use in observing the olfactory correlates of psychochemical patterns. My initial hope had been that Carter could dope out the rest for himself.

Obviously, at first he hadn't. But he apparently had had second thoughts when he later recalled the initial good days he had experienced on the suggested test diet. So he went back and carefully discovered for himself *why* he had felt so good at the beginning of the test. He found that he reacted either strongly positively or strongly negatively to many of the things he had been accustomed to eating, and that these reactions were correlated both with his days of energy and enthusiasm, and with his days of feeling "who cares?" and general pessimism.

He discovered that on those mornings he ate an orange, a few dates, and some walnuts for breakfast he not only would develop a headache, but would feel impatient and irritable, ready to jump on anyone who got in his way. And after such a breakfast he could detect no odors at all on the odor test—only a penetrating sensation in his nose and throat. At the other extreme, a breakfast of corned beef hash and bacon, one of his favorites, resulted in a dull, depressed feeling that might linger most of the day. After such a meal the odor test followed the pattern for slow oxidizers.

One might think that the obvious solution to Carter's wide shifts in reactions to food would be simply to "balance" the carbohydrates, fats, and types of protein in each meal so that no preponderant shift in metabolism would occur. However, this is far easier to suggest as a solution than to actually accomplish in action. In addition, Carter claimed that he rarely reacted to the same combination of foods in the same way. For example, a "balanced" breakfast of fruit juice, toast, poached eggs, and crisp bacon would one day push his oxidation rate way up, and on another day way down. In the first case the carbohydrates were too prominent for that particular day, while in the latter case the bacon and eggs slowed his oxidation rate too far down.

Part of the reason for this was in his previous day's nutrition. For example, a substantial dinner weighted toward the fat, purine-protein side (such as prime ribs with baked potato and butter) would call for an increase in the carbohydrates eaten next morning.

Predictably, other factors were also involved: the stress of the previous day and the anticipated difficulties of the coming day, the weather, possible infections, as well as allergies in certain seasons, and so on.

One must take into account the impossibility of accurately assessing these numerous variables. One must also take into account the practical exigencies of going about one's business instead of spending a lot of time and thought in planning what to eat or avoid. All these considerations demanded some relatively simple, manageable solution.

Before I resumed seeing him, Professor Carter himself had gone a long way toward solving his problem of attaining homeostatic stability. Noting from his odor responses that the most likely biochemical shift that occurred after eating was toward the fast side of the oxidation scale, he began to slant all meals a little toward the slow side: more fat and purine-protein, less carbohydrate. This plan had manifest drawbacks—often it threw him too far down in oxidation rate, with consequent depression and lack of energy, but he found it easier to correct this kind of error rather than to try to correct its opposite.

So I devised a modified miniature odor kit for him which he carried in his briefcase. When he felt "off" in any way, he relied on this test to provide clues for remedial action.

During an interview about a year or so later, Carter told me that "he had things pretty well under control." I then pushed a sheet of paper across my desk toward him on which I had jotted down a brief summary of his types of psychochemical response patterns.

CARTER, PAUL

Three personalities and their psychochemical bases:
1. *Wild, irritable, impatient, frequent headaches; very fast oxidation rate.*
2. *Sullen, depressed, hostile (also headaches but for a different reason); very slow oxidation rate.*
3. *Relaxed, optimistic, cooperative, pleasant; normal biochemical balance, no headaches.*

I wouldn't have dared do this if I hadn't known at the time that I was conversing with Paul Carter Number 3. He read the summary reflectively, and then pushed it back to me with a small smile.

Although I have used the phrase "homeostatic stability" in describing Carter's solution to his psychochemical variability, this really isn't an accurate term. For my experiences with Carter and with others like him lead me to believe that, once a person's homeostatic control systems lose their stabilizing capabilities, they don't seem to be completely reparable. Improved, yes; restored to normal, no.

Variable oxidizers, since their rates of energy production are unstable and unusually influenced by foods, physical and psychological stresses, and all the other variables, must learn by careful self-observation and experimentation what strategies of remedial action can help them achieve a more or less stable metabolism, with the consequent psychological and emotional composure that results from it. We will discuss in detail this problem and the nutritional measures one can take in coping with it in Chapter 4.

3

The Psychochemical Odor Test

The Psychochemical Odor Test is a unique means for knowing oneself both nutritionally and psychologically. In the nutritional context of the energy-producing processes occurring in the tissues, the test yields information that can be used in selecting the optimum foods for personality strength as well as in avoiding foods that will diminish that strength. This last statement defines the term "orthonutrition": the correct foods at the right time and in optimum amounts.

Psychologically, the test is useful primarily in providing clues for detecting the sources of inappropriate behavior (psychochemical responses) in everyday life. These range from mild depression, low energy, lack of confidence, inability to fix goals and carry through to success, sexual inadequacy, general anxiety, to serious mental and emotional disorders.

HOW THE ODOR TEST WORKS

Olfaction, the sense of smell, is a sense whose receptors are normally stimulated only by contact with airborne chemical substances. Apart from the many theories about how the nose does its work—none of which is completely acceptable—we do know that it is the most sensitive chemical detector known. It can detect concentrations of chemicals that are more than one hundred times weaker than the best scientific instruments (gas chromatographs).

Despite this great sensitivity, the sense of smell does not basically serve as a universal sensory detector in man as it does in other animals. Humans rarely rely on their sense of smell as a guide to action; they prefer to depend mainly upon visual rather than upon olfactory cues. This may indeed have a survival value, for it is well known that entirely different chemical substances may have similar or identical odors. There appears to be no simple and direct relationship between chemical composition and odor.

This fact lies at the foundation of the Psychochemical Odor Test. For what a given substance, say, dried liver powder or liver tablets, smells like to a given person depends predominantly upon the concentrations of certain nutritional biochemicals in that person's bloodstream and tissues, rather than upon the chemical composition of beef liver itself.

Accordingly, in test research subjects, one finds a wide range of answers to questions such as "Can you smell the tablets in this bottle?" "Can you say what they smell like?" "Is this a faint, mild, medium, or strong odor?"

However, even though various replies will be made by different persons for any given test substance, these descriptions fortunately fall into definite patterns or contexts. And, further, these patterns are related to and are characteristic of psychochemical types.

To illustrate the dependence of the sense of smell—of what a given substance such as dried liver smells like—upon one's own biochemistry, here is a simple experiment that can be self-convincing. Fill a small vial (one that is three or four inches high, with a top opening of about one inch—obtainable from any pharmacy) almost half full of beef liver tablets (obtainable at drug and health-food stores). After the tablets have been capped in the vial for an hour or so, remove the cap and briefly sniff the contents.

What you report the odor to be is, I have said, related to your own nutritional state. Let us assume, for simplicity, that you are a fast oxidizer, as Professor Carter frequently was. In this event you will most likely report that the contents of the vial have a faint sour odor. Other variants may be given, such as "spoiled," "musty," "moldy," or just "faint" without an aromatic adjective being mentioned.

Now—and here is the point of the test—swallow (with water) about eight or ten of the liver tablets, and retest the odor in about one-half hour. If the dose was large enough the odor will have changed, say from something like "sour" to perhaps "malt" or "wheat."

Repeated doses of the tablets will cause shifts in odor re-sponses until they register as "strong," "unpleasant," "like fertil-izer," or something of the sort. In the extreme case of a surfeit of liver tablets the nose will refuse to register an odor, and you won't be able to smell anything at all.

During such an experiment, the liver tablets haven't altered. The basic facts about the sense of smell are not only that there is no direct relationship between the chemical composition of what is being smelled and what it smells like, but that the reported odors are directly related to biochemical events occurring in the person doing the olfactory sensing.

In other words the sense of smell is a *projective sense* which attributes characteristics to objects that they do not "objectively" possess. Such a projective sense tells us more about the person doing the sensing than it does about the object being sensed.

You may wonder whether it was the liver tablets *as such*—a certain complex of biochemical substances—that were responsible for altering your sense of smell. The answer is "no," for the same pattern of changing odor responses to dehydrated beef liver can be caused by any combination of nutrients that will raise the blood sugar level and slow down the rate at which it is being broken down.

In addition to nutrients, some nonfood items can result in similar odor shifts: hormones (thyroid, androgens, and estrogens), as well as tranquilizers such as phenothiazines. In using the odor test, one should not test oneself for nutritional balance when complicating factors such as drugs and hormones may be involved.

I have used dried beef liver tablets to illustrate the shift in odor reports because we have found that the range of responses to them is qualitatively very great. For example, at the extreme end of the Fast Oxidizer Scale the test subject reports smelling nothing, but rather feeling a prickling sensation in the nose. This is the condition Professor Carter was in on those days he arrived at his laboratory "wild and sort of crazy, with a certain look that scares you."

Coming down the fast-oxidizing scale from very fast to very slow, the sequence of reported odors most often runs like this: from "penetrating or gassy" to "garbage," then "sour," then "faint food odor," "faint sweet," "chocolate," "malty," "cooking meat," "something rotting," "fertilizer," "burned," and finally "I can't smell anything at all."

HOW TO MAKE YOUR OWN
PSYCHOCHEMICAL ODOR KIT

Materials other than foods can be used for odor testing—aspirin, penicillin, antihistamines, etc. Although all of them reflect changes in metabolism, dehydrated foods appear to function best as test substances.

Since such a wide variety of potential materials is available, the problem of selecting the "best" test items is virtually unmanageable: an odor kit can be constructed in many different ways. The suggestions I have to offer have one paramount virtue: I have recorded and correlated literally thousands of odor profiles on research subjects, and while a person might respond with an occasional unique odor report to a given test sample, the inclusion of six *alternate* test materials is usually sufficient to fit even the most deviant research subject.

Again, you may obtain from your pharmacy, generally without cost, six plastic prescription-type vials that have caps that snap on and off *(don't* get vials with safety caps). They should be about 3½ inches high, with a diameter of about 1½ inches. The size of the test vial is of some importance; bottles with larger diameters will elicit different odor responses because they diminish the concentration of odor particles. The same is true for smaller vials. As silly as this may sound to a nonscientist, I have spent a great amount of time on this amorphous problem, including having a full-time research assistant exploring the problems of how best to achieve consistent test results with various shapes and sizes of containers, as well as with powdered test materials, liquid solutions of test materials, and simple uncoated seven-gram tablets of test substances.

Although work was started on these problems in 1950, and I have given considerable attention since then to developing a test that others can use with highly reliable results, I wouldn't care to give the impression that all of this effort has resulted in some kind of perfection. In many respects the problem is generally unmanageable by ordinary scientific quantitative standards. On the other hand, what has been developed is a pragmatic tool with high reliability that provides one with information that I know no other way of obtaining.

The odor test materials that are easily obtainable from health-food stores and yield results that are comparable to the specially formulated test substances that we use in our laboratory are the following:

1. *Food yeast (Torula) tablets* (not *brewer's yeast*).
2. *Whole-leaf dried alfalfa tablets.*
3. *Mammalian liver tablets. These may be pork, horse, goat, etc.; labels generally simply say "mammalian," and suppliers as a rule cannot give you more information.*
4. *Beef liver tablets.*
5. *Dehydrated cabbage-leaf tablets.*
6. *Citrus bioflavonoid complex tablets (composed of 150 mg. rose-hip vitamin C, 50 mg. rutin, 100 mg. citrus bioflavonoids (not lemon bioflavonoids), and—optional—hesperidin 50 mg.*°

The *order* in which these materials are listed is important, for they present an ascending scale of odor strength to a "normal" test subject. Often it is desirable to run the test on oneself or on a nonpatient just to check for this pattern.

In addition, however, each vial that one sniffs subtly influences one's response to the next in the series. The odor patterns given below take this fact into account, and the validity of scoring of the test depends in part upon running through the series of test vials from one to six. Each vial, therefore, should be clearly numbered, and each vial should be approximately one-third full of the appropriate test tablet.

° If you are unable to obtain the materials to make an odor kit—and there are vast areas in this country that contain no health-food stores—you may obtain a complete, *standardized* odor kit by ordering it by mail from Edom Laboratories, Inc., 860 Grand Blvd., Deer Park, N.Y. 11729. Phone (516) 586-2266.

THE USE OF THE PSYCHOCHEMICAL ODOR TEST IN
DETERMINING NUTRITIONAL BALANCE

The test is a self-administered one which yields scores on two scales, the Fast Oxidizer (FO) and the Slow Oxidizer (SO). The numerical *differences* between the scores of these two scales provide a clinical indication of the degree of imbalance in nutritional intake, allowing one to classify oneself as a fast oxidizer, a slow oxidizer, or a suboxidizer. On the other hand, a variable oxidizer is one whose scores on the test show frequent shifts from fast to slow to normal, etc., indicating erratic eating habits which can lead to psychological difficulties.

The scoring of the test is easy even for an eight-year-old. The highest possible score on either the FO or the SO scale is 72; the lowest possible score on either scale is 24. The difference between these scores allows one to classify oneself as either a slow or fast or suboxidizer.

SCORING YOURSELF ON THE
PSYCHOCHEMICAL ODOR TEST

The two scales on the test (which are given on pages 36–38), are what psychologists call "forced choice" scales: you must choose among the limited range of alternatives offered. If you look at the possible answers on the tests you will see that there are three groups offered for each test vial *(a, b, & c)*. Each of these groups contain several words which define a general "odor area" or "odor context." For example, Vial I, containing food yeast, under *a* asks you to choose among "pungent/musty/sour/fishy."

The adoption of the *odor context* conception came only after many years of effort to bring some kind of order into an area of seemingly impossible confusion. It was derived from computer

analysis of thousands of actual responses given by research subjects of each of the psychochemical types, to determine the fre-
quencies of their responses.

In scoring yourself on the test, it is best that you read over all
the choices offered for the vial you are about to test, so that you
can orient yourself into the odor context being offered.

Psychochemical Odor Test

FAST OXIDIZER SCALE

INSTRUCTIONS: Place a check mark before the group of al-
ternative odors for each of the numbered vials which closest approximates how you would describe the odor. In some cases none
of the alternatives will appear to you to be the right word, but
on many thousands of tests we have found that the alternatives
offered are the ones most likely to be selected by research subjects. Consequently, choose the group of descriptive words which
comes closest to what you would volunteer to say if you had a
free choice.

Vial I: Check either group a, b, or c.
a. _____ / pungent / musty / sour / fishy
b. _____ / grassy / nutty / grain / faint
c. _____ / burned / medicinal / spoiled / bitter

Vial II:

a. _____ / musty / grassy / moldy / sour
b. _____ / grain / grass / herbs / spice
c. _____ / bitter / liver / fertilizer / burned

Vial III:
a. _____ / garbage / mildew / pungent / earthy
b. _____ / yeast / grass / tea / grain
c. _____ / liver / bitter / fertilizer / pungent

Vial IV:
a. _____ / bad food / musty / sour / faint
b. _____ / yeast / grain / sweet / faint
c. _____ / bitter / barnyard / liver / burned

Vial V:
a. _____ / strong vegetable / sour / spoiled / faint
b. _____ / fruit / honey / grain / spice
c. _____ / burned / bitter / liver / spoiled

Vial VI:
a. _____ / faint / sour / garbage / pungent
b. _____ / tea / fruit / honey / spice
c. _____ / rotten / liver / bitter / burned

SLOW OXIDIZER SCALE

INSTRUCTIONS: Repeat the procedure described for record-ing your reactions to each of the six vials as you have just done for the "Fast Oxidizer Scale." The reason for retesting on an al-ternate scoring system is that the *differences* in your responses to the two different scales yield a highly reliable index of your psychochemical type.

Vial I: Check either group a, b, or c.
a. _____ / burned / medicinal / spoiled / faint
b. _____ / herbs / molasses / yeast / alfalfa
c. _____ / moldy / sour / bad food / pungent

Vial II:
a. _____ / liver / burned / barnyard / rotten
b. _____ / alfalfa / straw / wheat / tea
c. _____ / pungent / spoiled / musty / sour

Vial III:
a. _____ / bitter / fertilizer / burned / spoiled
b. _____ / food odor / hay / musty / faint
c. _____ / sour / spoiled / pungent / garbage

Vial IV:
a. _____ / strong liver / bitter / faint / fertilizer
b. _____ / straw / food odor / liver / grass
c. _____ / pungent / sour / herbs / faint

Vial V:
a. _____ / bad food / burned / fertilizer / faint
b. _____ / grass / hay / vegetable / grain
c. _____ / moldy / sour / garbage / faint

Vial VI:
a. _____ / bitter / burned / medicinal / rotten
b. _____ / pungent / sweet / hay / faint
c. _____ / sour / herbs / yeast / tea

The following is a summary of the scores which define fast oxidizers, slow oxidizers, and suboxidizers.

FAST OXIDIZERS

Each a selection that you make counts 12 points.
Each b selection that you make counts 8 points.
Each c selection that you make counts 4 points.

If you were to select all *a* choices, your total score would be 72, which is the maximum, and is *generally* recorded only by very disturbed individuals.° However, the *average* score for fast oxidizers is 60 on the Fast Oxidizer Scale, while it is 32 on the Slow Oxidizer Scale. You are a fast oxidizer if the difference between your scores on the two scales is 28 (60 minus 32 equals 28).

SLOW OXIDIZERS

The scoring system for both scales is the same: each *a* selection counts 12; each *b* selection counts 8, while each *c* selection counts 4. If you were to select all *a* odor contexts your score would be 72, most likely indicating serious psychological and emotional difficulties.° In that event you would have selected (most probably) all *c* selections on the Fast Oxidizer Scale, yielding a 48-point difference, which is the maximum. Scores in these extreme ranges are generally only found in emotionally and mentally disturbed individuals.° However, the *average* score for slow oxidizers is 60 on the Slow Oxidizer Scale and 32 on the Fast Oxidizer Scale. You are a slow oxidizer if the difference between your scores on the two scales is 28.

SUBOXIDIZERS AND NORMALS

The same method of scoring for these types is used; both suboxidizers and normals will score 48 on both the Fast Oxidizer and Slow Oxidizer scales, resulting in 0 (zero) difference between the two scales.

° The chance of a "normal" individual recording a very high score is less than one in a hundred. Some of such cases are included in later chapters.

The numbers given in the foregoing discussion are for purposes of defining the way the test is constructed. In practice, however, there is a range of variance for classifying a patient into one of the groups. For example, an individual who showed a 6-point difference between the scales, rather than a 0-point difference, would be termed "normal." The rule to use when scores don't fit ideal patterns is to judge the patient's status by whether his score is closer to "normal" (0 difference) or approaches the extreme limit of abnormality (48 points). In this manner one can estimate what the appropriate therapy should be. This is the best that can be done in what is essentially a clinical situation: you are classified according to which way the scores tend to fall, toward normal, slow, or fast oxidation. In practice, however, one rarely finds borderline cases. People who are depressed, anxious, hostile, etc. virtually always fit into the basic patterns described above.

The Psychochemical Odor Test cannot identify normal individuals who are suboxidizers; these are people whose biochemical balance is "normal," but who experience "psychological" problems such as fatigue, apathy, disinterest, and so on. Diet surveys (covering at least a week's food intake) generally show that the suboxidizer is not getting an optimum amount of all of the nutrients he needs to feel "normal." Blood tests of hemoglobin and total carbon dioxide may help. But I have found that a good dietary survey and analysis leads to the quickest results in recovery.

The following is a typical example of how a person being tested responds to the six odor test vials.

The patient in question was a thirty-three-year-old life-insurance salesman who had been a member of what his company called the "Million Dollar Round Table" for three consecutive years. That is, he sold a million dollars' worth of life insurance each year for three years, which I gather is no easy matter.

The following year he sold around $700,000 worth, but the next year was a disaster. He said, "I worked as hard as I could, but I just didn't seem to have it—whatever that it is. I had the leads but I couldn't close the deals. I sold less than $500,000 worth of life insurance. And the way things are going this year, I'm about ready to quit. I've got to the place where I simply don't give a damn about life insurance—or about anything else, for that matter."

He had come to see me because, ironically, I had been a client of his during one of his million-dollar years. I had got to know him in a casual way. When I first met him he seemed very much "alive," talked easily but quietly, and sort of gave one the impression that here was a person one simply seemed to "know," even though I'd only talked with him an hour or so.

But now, three years later, his sparkle was gone. He was simply flat, and his voice pattern and general manner suggested weariness—hardly the image one ought to project in trying to sell anything, much less life insurance.

These were his answers to the six odor test materials:

    I. Food yeast: burned.
    II. Alfalfa: burned.
   III. Mammalian liver: fertilizer.
   IV. Beef liver: bitter.
    V. Dried cabbage: bad food.
   VI. Bioflavonoids: burned.

If you will check these answers on the Fast and Slow Oxidizer scales (pages 36 to 38) you will see that he scored the minimum (24) on the Fast Oxidizer Scale and the maximum (72) on the Slow Oxidizer Scale—a difference of 48 points.

These scores reflect a very slow rate of converting food into energy, which was the problem of Roy Canfield. Also, the causes of Canfield's decline were very much like those of this life insurance man's decline: biochemical erosion. They each worked too long, too hard, without knowing that they were burning themselves out.

The psychological crises illustrated by each of these cases could have been prevented had they each possessed a Psychochemical Odor kit together with the dietary knowledge necessary to correct their nutritional inadequacies.

I now suggested to this young man that he see his physician as soon as possible for a thorough examination. I also provided him with an odor test kit, plus detailed nutritional information telling him what to do under the varying conditions the test might indicate. I told him to see his physician because undetected or unsuspected illnesses—diabetes, tuberculosis, etc.—can alter odor test scores. In general, when nutritional changes do not result in the expected changes of odor test scores, one must look to something other than nutritional biochemistry for an explanation.

He made an appointment to see me again in one month, at which time he told me that, although he'd had to have a badly infected tooth extracted, the doctor's report was essentially satisfactory. Clinically he seemed improved, and the difference between his scores on the Psychochemical Odor Test had dropped from 48 to 36.

Since we appeared to be on the right track, I told him he need not bother to see me again as long as he was improving. About a year later he phoned, saying that he was in the neighborhood and would just like to stop by to say "hello." He sounded very good, and this should have warned me.

He said a little bit more than "hello"; he sold me double my previous insurance coverage, which I didn't think I needed. But he assured me that I did, and that my cash reserve on my present policy would take care of the payments for a long time. And, though *I* was convinced I couldn't afford it and didn't need it, I bought it anyway. I guess this is a good illustration of salesmanship.

4

What Is Orthonutrition?

"Correct nutrition" is only applicable to an individual, not to a group (such as "infants" or "adults" or "the elderly"), who might be judged to be "adequately nourished" or "undernourished" by some statistical averaging yardstick. For example, there are the "recommended daily allowances" offered by the National Research Council. But the assumption which underlies the notion of recommended daily allowances is that the population as a whole is relatively uniform in biochemical makeup and that nutritional needs are about the same for everyone.

Consequently, I use the term "orthonutrition" to draw attention to the need to recognize the importance of *individual* nutritional requirements that are simply overlooked by dieticians and physicians generally. The prefix "ortho" is from the Greek meaning "straight." This prefix has come to have several usages, and the meaning it carries in "orthonutrition" is "correct."

Even if you make sure that your daily food intake meets the suggested U.S. government recommendations it may still be possible that you are inadequately nourished by orthonutritional standards. There is a large and growing body of nutritional research which reveals wide variations in biochemical needs among those who *appear* to be "normal, average, healthy persons." My standards are not something I personally thought up.

44

For example, consider the following ranges of concentrations of several important constituents of "normal" human blood:[*]

	Range—mg., %
Glucose	*84–125*
Glycogen	*1.2–16.2*
Lactic acid	*0–41.0*
Pyruvic acid	*0.4–2.0*
Adenosine triphosphate	*31–57*

I have selected these particular blood variables because they are all involved directly in the energy-producing activities of the tissues. All five of them can be increased or decreased by selecting the orthodiet—the individualized diet—that you and you alone will benefit most by. In my research, I've never encountered *anyone* who was acting at his full potential capacity.

The last item on the brief list above, adenosine triphosphate, is the principal source of energy in the body. And yet, in the bloodstreams of some allegedly normal, healthy persons there is almost twice as much adenosine triphosphate as there is in the bloodstreams of other normal persons. This important substance is *increased* through orthonutrition, with the expected positive consequent changes in personality and behavior.

An adequate description of adenosine triphosphate would require a basic course in biochemistry. The important thing to know, however, is that it is the principal energy carrier of the body. Adenosine triphosphate—or, as the biochemist calls it, ATP—is produced in the cells of the tissues by the oxidation of blood sugar (glucose) and its intermediates, as well as by the oxidation of protein and fat. The production of ATP depends basically upon the availability of nutrients in one's diet: the purine

[*] Williams, Roger J., *Biochemical Individuality* (New York: Wiley, 1963), page 52.

base adenine and the mineral phosphate. It also depends upon carbohydrates, protein, and all of the vitamins and minerals required for the utilization of food, as well as the action of several hormones (such as insulin and epinephrine). Although the body can and does synthesize some of these materials (such as adenine), additional amounts obtained from the diet are of added value.

ATP production depends not only upon what one eats but also upon one's genetic (hereditary) biochemical makeup. All of the energy-producing systems in the body are controlled by enzymes, the protein catalysts formed by living cells from nutrients obtained from one's diet. One's inherited genetic code directs the manufacture of enzymes. Consequently, one's maximum potential for activity of any kind is built right into the cells of the body. Through self-knowledge and appropriate dietary behavior one may be able to reach this potential, but one cannot alter it. The ultimate level of performance remains hereditarily determined and biological.

What I am discussing in this book is the role of biological energy production in personality strength. Such energy production is the absolute basis from which we must *start*. My interest is in teaching people how to know themselves *biochemically*. But it would be a gross oversimplification to say that achieving one's maximum personality potential through orthonutrition is the equivalent of achieving the "good life." Indeed, in rare cases, achieving one's maximum personality potential can be about the worst thing that could happen, as we will see in Chapter 5.

Still, in my view, the effects of negative life experiences definitely need not be obstacles to becoming a strong person. Are there any lasting effects of, say, a wretched childhood, which would make it impossible for the victim to achieve his or her maximum energy output potential?

In the psychological sense, the answer is "no," and this is a carefully considered reply based upon the study of hundreds of cases with this kind of problem. What *typically* happens to an individual who is carrying a heavy load of accumulated psychological insults is that as his or her energy level increases the emotional load becomes lighter. In general, strong personalities simply don't look back. Weak persons dwell on the troubles they've had, which they believe have ruined their lives. For example, they put the blame for their failures on overly strict parents, broken homes, uncaring, unloving mothers. "I was an unwanted child," a young woman told me, "and nobody since has shown the least interest in whether I lived or died." I ran a diet survey on her and found that she was living on yogurt, bean sprouts, sesame seeds, and meditation.

These foods are good, of course, in their proper contexts. And meditation no doubt was of help to her in the pitiful biochemical condition we found her to be in. But within three months after being put on her orthonutritional program she volunteered the remark that her parents were "really good people" who did the best they could for her and her two younger brothers under very hard conditions. "I now feel very sorry for them and what they went through to raise a family."

On the other hand, I must add that lasting biochemical damage can result from early nutritional deprivation. Damage of this kind is usually undetectable—it may be quite subtle; consequently our approach to every research patient is to ignore this problem and try to advance the individual as far as we can, regardless of what early nutritional deprivations may have done for his or her potential growth.

In general, patients who have been placed on the orthonutritional program change their perceptions of themselves, with the consequence that they—in a sense—leave behind them their "old selves." Their former selves may have been largely a collection of psychological failures (or "hangups"). This is very often the case, and, to the extent that it is true, the patients' newly acquired personality strength could be said to have eliminated former psychological blocks. After they've been treated, they are still the "same people," but only in the sense of name, date of birth, social security number, and so on. Their perceptions of themselves change because they now perceive a *different personality*. With new strength come new goals; they see relationships differently; their world takes on new meaning in terms of the way they now evaluate themselves, particularly among the people with whom they've been associated, and they look at both their past and what their future may be in almost entirely different terms.

In short, then, they are *not* the "same people" if one defines a person in terms of how he or she thinks, feels, and acts. We will return to this most interesting subject in a later chapter, with case histories of the kinds of personality changes one observes in persons who begin to function at a much higher biochemical level.

I would like to return to the question raised earlier, namely, the relationship between purely psychological problems and those that appear to be psychological but actually orginate in personality weaknesses due to poor biochemical functioning. How can these be identified and separated?

Approximately 80 percent of our research patients with alleged "psychological problems" had previously been treated unsuccessfully with some form of talk therapy (psychotherapy). It is my view that it would be better for the patient and for the therapist to *first* treat the patient orthonutritionally for at least six months, and then evaluate the patient from a strictly psychological point of view to see what problems remain. In other words, a problem may be psychological if one can eliminate the possibility that it is biochemical. The opposite approach—that the problem may be biochemical if it can't be handled psychologically—may be valid. But in my view it is the wrong approach. Wrong because psychotherapy itself is lengthy, expensive, and for the most part (depending upon the nature of the problem) of limited success. It seems obvious to me that one should try the quickest, cheapest, and basically essential approach first.

To some degree, there are rules and cues a person can use to tell whether he or she is functioning at his or her maximum biochemical capacity. The following list allows one to evaluate quickly one's *present* status. Your diet is *adequate* (but not necessarily *optimum*) if you:

1. *Have interest and enthusiasm for much of what you do.*
2. *Pay attention to personal hygiene and appearance.*
3. *Are not gaining or losing weight.*
4. *Are not hungry between meals.*
5. *Do not experience mid-morning or mid-afternoon energy letdowns.*
6. *Are not exhausted at the end of a day's work.*
7. *Are not still tired when the alarm clock rings in the morning (assuming you've had adequate sleep).*
8. *In addition to these seven cues for nutritional adequacy, additional considerations must be made for women (pages 58–61).*

On the other hand, your diet is probably *inadequate* if you:

1. *Have little or no interest in either your work or recreation.*
2. *Feel the need frequently to seek stimulants such as coffee, alcohol, tobacco, or other drugs in order to "enjoy yourself."*
3. *Have little or no appetite or interest in food, or the opposite, want to eat junk food frequently.*
4. *Have little interest in personal cleanliness or appearance: hair*

dirty, fingernails dirty and uncared for, toenails untrimmed, teeth not brushed regularly, clothes dirty, strong body odor due to infrequent bathing.

5. *Feel "down"—tired and listless—most of the time.*
6. *Are "touchy," irritable, and tend to feel friendless, ignored, and unappreciated.°*

The problem of reaching one's maximum capability must be approached on a trial-error basis. First let us assume that you score "normal" on the Psychochemical Odor Test, meaning that your biochemical balance of the intake of the various food groups is satisfactory. Then let us assume that you are a suboxidizer, capable of creating more energy than you are now doing.

Now you adopt the orthodiet recommended for suboxidizers. But before you do this you should make a daily list for one week of your interests, attitudes toward phases of your life (such as yourself and your job), as well as your activities—what you do with your spare time.

Such a list is really necessary, for I have observed radical changes in the behavior and attitudes of patients when they themselves were unaware that they had changed at all. Their failure to recognize changes may be attributed to the fact that we live unilaterally, so to speak. We experience ourselves continuously. But we don't contrast or compare ourselves with "another self"—namely the person we were two weeks ago—and what that person was thinking, feeling, and doing.

Let me give you an illustration of this phenomenon. In interviewing patients I write down the exact words that they use to describe their problems. I had a language professor tell me in our first interview, "I'm so exhausted by noon that I don't see

---

°As in the cues for nutritional adequacy, special attention must be given to poorly nourished women. This is discussed in detail on pages 58–61.

how I'm going to get through the day. I never think of tomorrow, for I can't imagine that I can endure what's in store for me."

At his next appointment one month later he said, "There's been no change, no improvement. I just face it from day to day." I asked him if he was doing anything outside of his teaching, say, in the way of recreation. "Oh, that," he said. "Yes, I've started this last week playing a little tennis after school to keep my mind off correcting student papers. I don't know whether it helps or not."

The following month he again said, "I don't think I'm getting anywhere. If I can survive this last month before vacation begins, I'll be lucky. My wife and I are planning a trip to Europe for two months, which I hope will put me back on my feet."

Well, of course it is obvious to anyone observing this transition that the professor not only landed on his feet but had hit the ground moving if not running. He sent me postcards from England, France, Italy, and Spain, and each had some reference to the trip being "tiring." Yet this intelligent man had never before even *considered* taking a vacation away from home—much less a two-month tour of Europe.

The following is a list of some basic characteristics of one's behavior that are variable and that reflect increases in energy that one might not think significant:

1. *Time of arising.*
2. *Attitude toward what one plans to do during the day.*
3. *The care with which one grooms oneself.*
4. *The attention one gives to selecting the appropriate attire for the day.*
5. *The time it takes to do all this—to get going.*
6. *One's plans for the evening: is it just TV and bed or some activity that is culturally and intellectually rewarding?*

Here are before-and-after sample lists from a married (twenty-five-year-old) woman (no children):

BEFORE ORTHONUTRITION PROGRAM STARTED:

1. *"I get up around nine or nine-thirty. My husband leaves for work at seven-thirty, and makes his own breakfast."*
2. *"Today I have no plans except to get something for dinner and have dinner ready around six, when my husband gets home from work."*
3. *"In the morning after I arise I spend about two hours over coffee and a sweet roll while I glance at the morning paper."*
4. *"I put all the dishes to soak, and then get ready to go to the store. I skip lunch but have some pizza later in the afternoon."*
5. *"I most frequently go around the shops in the shopping center, just to kill time after I've bought my groceries."*
6. *"I get home around four or so and begin dinner, and after dinner we watch television until eleven or so, when we go to bed."*

AFTER FOUR MONTHS ON HER ORTHODIET:

1. *"Up at six forty-five to make sure my husband gets a good breakfast. After he leaves for work I do all the dishes."*
2. *"Must wash and set my hair. Going to an eleven-o'clock meeting of a club I used to belong to but had dropped out of—I don't remember just why I dropped out. After the meeting we will all have lunch."*
3. *"Going shopping with two friends. I just realized a few days ago how tacky almost everything I've been wearing looks."*
4. *"Home by four to fix early dinner, because I have to be at class—I've enrolled in a creative writing class at the Community College—by seven. The class meets once a week on Wednesdays for a three-hour period, and each week we have to submit a written assignment."*
5. *"We've quit watching TV regularly. I have homework to do and I have to read quite a bit of material—English literature—because I*

haven't read anything it seems for years. I really don't understand how I lost interest in reading. I was an English major in college."

This woman's original lifestyle was not unusual. But just because one frequently encounters such "half-alive" behavior does not make it acceptable. It wasn't acceptable to her. She entered our program because she felt she was "vegetating": she had no interests, and each day was "just one more day."

Were her behavior changes important? *She* thought the changes were just what she wanted: new energy, new interests, renewed contact with neglected friends—in short, she became alive and was beginning to become a participant rather than an indifferent and bored spectator in the world.

A complete diet list for obtaining maximum nutrient intake includes the following foods:

1. *Four different types of protein.*
2. *At least two different types of carbohydrates.*
3. *Two different types of fats.*
4. *Both water-soluble and fat-soluble vitamins.*
5. *Bulk minerals.*
6. *Trace elements.*
7. *Vegetable fiber.*

At first reading this may sound complicated beyond attainment. But I will reduce the complex types (which one really doesn't need to remember in detail) by restating them in terms of food we are all familiar with.

The word "protein" actually involves a far wider range of foods than merely four types. There is a greater diversity in the chemical composition of proteins than there is in the composition of any other group of nutritionally important foods. Fortunately we can ignore many of these complexities when it comes to choosing a diet.

The first thing to know about protein foods is that they are composed of amino acids, eight of which are essential and must be present in a given food (or combination of foods) *at the same time* in order to meet the needs of the body.

Foods that contain all of these basic amino acids are said to be "complete proteins." All of them are contained only in meat, fish, seafoods, fowl, eggs, cheese, and milk. Such protein foods are *complete* because they replace daily body protein losses. You will notice that the foods I have listed are all of animal origin. However, these eight amino acids can be obtained from the right combination of vegetables, with each providing two or three of the essential ones. This procedure, however, is far too complicated and exacting to provide the protein needs of the average individual untrained in nutritional biochemistry. By that, I do not mean to give the impression that a college course in nutritional biochemistry is necessary if you wish to be a vegetarian. I *do* mean that, if you choose to be a vegetarian, you must become familiar with the amino-acid contents of what you eat, and make sure that your choices will add up to a complete protein. In addition, no vegetable contains the important vitamin B_{12}; so a vegetarian must take a daily supplement of this vitamin. In short, the life of a vegetarian is a very complicated one if that person wishes to achieve the goal of orthonutrition. I personally could not do this. I am unwilling to spend the time it takes to analyze what I eat, and to make sure I am on the right track.

Unless you are willing to spend the time and vexations involved in balancing amino-acid combinations three times a day, you can't add animal foods, such as milk, cheese, and eggs to such a "vegetarian diet" and claim to be a vegetarian. It is sheer self-delusion to call oneself a "vegetarian" and then rely on animal sources for one's protein. From a practical point of view, if one wishes to achieve orthonutrition, complete proteins from animal sources are essential. As we shall see, foods like milk and eggs are of limited orthonutritional value for some psychochemical types but useful for others. This will be discussed in the following pages.

In addition to their amino-acid contents, some protein foods contain another class of nutrients called "nucleoproteins." These are foods which contain purine and pyrimidine bases, which play essential roles in the energy-producing systems of the tissues. By far the most important of these from the energy point of view is a purine base called adenine, which is a constituent of ATP. Adenine also plays a part in many other important components of the body, but a discussion of these is beyond the scope and intention of this book.

While adenine can be synthesized in the body (from CO_2, formate, aspartic acid, glycine, and glutamine), the body also utilizes the adenine contained in protein foods. "Nucleoproteins" contain the principal bases adenine, guanine, cytosine, and thymine. Their availability in the diet makes a critical difference in one's total personality strength. The most important of these bases from our point of view are adenine and guanine: the biochemist calls these purines. The following tables list some common foods with high purine content and some with medium.

FOODS WITH HIGH PURINE CONTENT

anchovies	liver
brains	kidney
meat gravies or soups	sweetbreads
heart	mussels
herring	sardines
caviar (any type)	meat extracts

FOODS WITH MODERATE PURINE CONTENT°

meat, any kind	*spinach*
turkey	*lentils*
chicken	*yeast*
fish	*whole-grain bread*
shrimp	*and cereals*
scallops	*beans*
oysters	*peas*
crabs	*mushrooms*
asparagus	*peanuts*
cauliflower	

I have now mentioned three of the four types of important protein foods: complete proteins, incomplete proteins, and proteins that are good sources of nucleoproteins. In looking over the above lists, you will find that several *incomplete* proteins, such as yeast and beans, are good sources of nucleoproteins.

The fourth—and last—type of proteins are complete proteins that contain the eight essential amino acids but do not contain nucleoproteins of any value (0–15 mg. per 100 gm. of food). I call these "neutral protein foods." *That* is where milk, cheese, and eggs come in.

From the viewpoint of orthonutrition, then, one should select one's proteins by two criteria: first, is it a complete protein? and second, is it a good source of nucleoproteins as well as being a complete protein? If you examine the lists of foods carefully, you will see that there is a very great range of foods to choose from that meet these criteria.

As I have mentioned, the Psychochemical Odor Test is the key

° The purine contents in these lists range from 150 mg. to 1,000 mg. per 100 grams of food. Since individual foods vary unpredictably within each group, one must accept averages.

to selecting the proteins best for you. For example, if you are a slow oxidizer, what I have called "neutral protein foods" would be your best choice. But, since this is a limited group of foods, some items from the "moderate purine" list, particularly chicken and fish, can be added.

If you are a fast oxidizer, your protein foods should be selected from the high and moderate purine lists. One must keep in mind that some of the foods on the moderate purine lists are *not* complete proteins: asparagus, cauliflower, spinach, yeast, whole-grain cereals and bread, beans, peas, peanuts, mushrooms. I have emphasized this fact because I have found that people tend to *assume* that if a food is a good source of nucleoproteins it is also a complete protein.

If you are a suboxidizer, however, you are fortunate, for you can eat any of the foods I have mentioned. Even so, a suboxidizer is a person who is not creating all of the energy he is capable of, so he or she should make most protein choices from the high and moderate purine lists.

And, finally, if your chemical balance is unstable and you are therefore a variable oxidizer, you must solve your protein intake on a day-to-day or even a meal-to-meal basis.

While most of the variable oxidizers I have studied have gradually been able to stabilize their systems through regular use of the Psychochemical Odor Test, so that they can eat "normally"—that is, choose whatever foods they want to eat—some must rely on the odor tests daily before planning their meals.

How does one determine one's optimum protein intake?

I have found that a sufficiently generous amount is about one gram per 2.2 pounds of body weight. This formula can be reduced to a simple rule: divide your ideal weight—what you think you would like to weigh—by the number 15. This number 15 is based upon the average protein content of all complete proteins. The result you obtain is the ounces of cooked meat and/or fish that will satisfy your protein needs for a day.

If you weigh, say, 150 pounds, and you divide this by 15, you will come up with 10. This means you should have about 3½ ounces of complete protein for each of three meals. One cup of milk or one medium-size egg approximates one ounce of meat, and when I say "cooked meat" I am referring to *lean* meat; not, say, a fatty pork or beef roast.

After you have determined your optimum protein intake, and computed or estimated its caloric value, the remaining number of necessary calories should be derived from whole-grain cereals (in bread or breakfast cereals, etc.), raw and cooked vegetables, and fresh fruit.° The sample menus given in Chapter 7 will spell this problem out in detail.

I have mentioned earlier (page 49) that special considerations in dietary choices apply to women. These concern the menstrual cycle and its relation to optimum nutrition.

One of the first signs of inadequate and incorrect nutrition is failure to menstruate regularly.† Other symptoms very commonly experienced by women with biochemical insufficiencies and imbalances are premenstrual tension, cramps, fluid retention, breast enlargement and tenderness, depression, fatigue, and general irritability.

In studying these problems in a large number of research patients we have found that most of these complaints can be minimized or eliminated in otherwise healthy women. Consider the following typical case history:

° The caloric values of foods are obtainable from any of the many paperback books available at newstands and bookstores.

† This statement is true. But of course there are many other possible causes for menstrual irregularities besides failure to provide nutrients for hormone production. A woman must consult her physician to rule out all such possibilities.

Mrs. K., a twenty-eight-year-old married woman (no children), volunteered for the research program, reporting the following symptoms:

Beginning about four to five days before she expected her period she began to feel "all dragged out." A day or so later she began to have spells of crying "over nothing at all." Three days before the expected period she noted that she couldn't get her feet into her regular shoes. Both her ankles and her feet were enlarged and "puffy." In addition, she couldn't get into her regular sheath-type dresses, and felt full and bloated all over. It hurt to wear a bra. The day preceding her period she said her cramps were so severe that she had to stay in bed.

On the other hand, during the last fourteen days of her menstrual cycle she usually felt "real good." She played some tennis and golf, but nothing strenuous or on a regular basis.

She was given an odor test kit and asked to record her scores every morning for a month. She was also asked to record what she ate for meals and snacks during this period.

Here is a summary of her odor test patterns during her menstrual cycle:

Two days after the end of her period she scored 4 points fast (52 on the fast scale; 48 on the slow scale). This is a "normal" reading, but indicates a tendency to fast oxidation of food.

Six days after the end of her period she scored 4 points slow (52 slow, 48 fast). This is still a "normal" score, but the eight-point shift from 4 fast to 4 slow in a matter of four days *might* be significant.

Twelve days after the end, and two days before the start of her next period, she scored 24 points slow (64 on the slow scale; 40 on the fast scale).

This radical shift from 4 fast to 24 slow coincided with the onset of all of the premenstrual discomforts and real suffering she generally experienced.

We have discovered through trial-and-error nutritional therapy that if one could maintain a normal Psychochemical Odor
Test score throughout the first fourteen days of the menstrual
cycle, the unwanted symptoms of fatigue, depression, crying,
cramps, etc. could be greatly reduced, and frequently eliminated. Thus a woman who keeps her ideal psychochemical balance
throughout the entire twenty-eight days would maintain her total personality strength. Menstruation now becomes little more
than a nuisance.

To accomplish this goal requires special attention to what one
eats and what vitamin-mineral supplements one takes. In the
case history given above, the following are the nutritional
changes that were made to counteract the slowing down of the
oxidation rate as the time for ovulation approached:

1. *As long as the patient scored 4 points fast her meals should be selected from the lists (pages 119-120) for fast oxidizers (4-16).*
2. *When her odor test scores had switched to 4 points slow, her food
   was to be selected from the lists (pages 125 ff.) for slow oxidizers
   (4-16).*
3. *When her score reached 24 slow (S-64; F-40), her meals were to be
   selected from the lists (pages 126 ff.) of foods for slow oxidizers
   (16-32).*

Changes in dietary supplements corresponded to the changes
in what she was eating:

1. *When she scored 4 points fast she took the fast oxidizer supplement (page 65) for those scoring 4-16 fast on the odor test.*
2. *When she scored 4 points slow she took the slow oxidizer supplement for those scoring 4-16 slow (page 64).*
3. *When her premenstrual score reached its maximum, 24 points
   slow, she took the supplement for those scoring 16-32 on the odor
   test.*

As she followed this plan, the shift in her biochemical balance from two days after her last period to four days before beginning her new period was not significant. She began the twenty-eight-day cycle at 4 points fast, and the morning of the day her period began her score was 4 points slow. Both scores were thus normal. Compare these figures with her before-treatment scores of 4 points fast (beginning) and 24 points slow at the start of her period.

What impressed her the most was "no cramps!" Also she reported no crying, a little fatigue, and some fluid retention.

Obviously she did well, but I felt that some adjustments in both diet and vitamin-mineral supplementation could produce the result I always aimed for: the approach of menstruation should not be apparent. No physical and emotional changes that generally signal the onset of menstruation should occur. This goal *can* be accomplished, and you can do it for yourself.

I find it troubling that it is virtually *impossible* to give full, technical answers to questions on nutrition and still hold the reader's attention. When things sound complicated, the average person thinks "this is not for me. I can live without all this junk fouling up my life." So I have to try to tell you how to make an atomic device while watching TV? Well, I can't do it.

Earlier I mentioned "two types of fat." This is something of an oversimplication. The fats in food are almost as complex as the proteins. But, for our purposes, there are basically two types. One of these is the *poly*unsaturated fats such as soybean oil and corn oil, whereas simple "unsaturated" fats such as olive oil do not count as essential fats. The polyunsaturated fats *are essential* in the diet. Fortunately the body's daily requirements are easily met by using soybean- or corn-oil margarines or salad dressings. Some prefer safflower oil to corn or soybean oil. Safflower oil happens to be more unsaturated than the others, but the difference isn't significant. It comes down to a matter of taste.

The other type of fat is animal fat. This is essential in the diet as the carrier of fat-soluble vitamins such as D, E, A, and K. Laboratory animals whose nutritional needs are similar to ours do poorly when their fat is cut to 20 percent of the diet; do best when it is 30 to 40 percent. Most nutritional scientists would prefer diets that do not contain more than 30 percent; some prefer less. (I am here referring to diets for normal persons: normal blood pressure, etc.)

The following summation lists the principal foods that have an *adverse* effect upon fast and slow oxidizers—and should be used rarely:

FAST OXIDIZERS—FOODS TO AVOID

1. *Proteins: milk, buttermilk, yogurt, cottage cheese, low-fat cheese (such as homemade soufflés), fish (except herring, sardines, anchovies, tuna, and salmon).*
2. *Carbohydrates: pastries, candies, fruit, jams, jellies, ice cream, soft drinks, potatoes, macaroni, spaghetti, bread or cereals (any kind except cooked oatmeal).*
3. *Salads: lettuce, green peppers, onions, tomatoes, radishes, cabbage, pickles, cucumbers (celery and carrot sticks excepted; no carrot or celery juice, such as that made in a blender).*
4. *Miscellany: spicy sauces (containing any kind of pepper), catsup, artificially sweetened soft drinks, coffee (decaffeinated allowed), tea, beer, wine, or any other alcoholic beverage.*

SLOW OXIDIZERS—FOODS TO AVOID

1. *Proteins: foods with high purine content such as liver, kidney, etc. (generally, all foods with high or medium purine content as listed above).*
2. *Vegetables: avocado, beans, peas, lentils, cauliflower, spinach, asparagus, potato casserole made with cream, milk, and cheddar cheese.*

3. *Fats: lard and butter should be replaced with corn, soy, or safflower oil for both salad dressings and butter substitutes.*
4. *Beverages: any alcoholic drink that exceeds 12 percent alcohol by volume. Coffee and tea are acceptable.*
5. *General: any concentrated sweet, or any concentrated fat (saturated) food.*

Finally, you should note that the foods to avoid for fast oxidizers are the foods that are recommended for slow oxidizers, and that the foods to avoid for slow oxidizers are those recommended for fast oxidizers.

Vitamin-mineral supplements are necessary for *both* fast and slow oxidizers. The formulas below have been tested on several thousand patients. When accompanied by the appropriate diet, larger quantities are not needed in most cases. However, the higher one's score on the Psychochemical Odor Test, the larger is one's need for added supplements. (When I mention one's "score" on the test I am referring to the point excess of one scale over the other. A fast oxidizer with a score of 10, consequently, has scored 10 points more on the Fast Oxidizer Scale than he has on the Slow Oxidizer Scale. Thus one is "10 points fast" or "10 points slow" and so on.)

Consequently, the tablets or capsules should be so formulated that one may take either the basic formula *or* multiples of it— say, two to four times the amount given below. The quantity you take is determined by your Psychochemical Test Score. For example, if one is a fast (or slow) oxidizer, with a score which is 10 points or more in favor of either the fast or slow side (38 points on either scale, where "normal" is 48), the quantities listed below (the basic intake) should, within a month for most cases, cause a drop in your score of 5 or more points. However, if your score does not decrease, then double the amount of vitamins and minerals you have been taking. Thus, by continued checking of your odor test scores, you can ultimately adjust your vitamin-mineral intake to the optimum level for you.

BASIC SLOW OXIDIZER SUPPLEMENT

Total Daily Amount		*Each Capsule to Contain*	
Vitamin A	15,000 I.U.	Vitamin A	5,000 I.U.
(fish liver oil)			
Niacin	75 mg.	Niacin	25 mg.
Vitamin B₁	30 mg.	Vitamin B₁	10 mg.
Vitamin B₂	30 mg.	Vitamin B₂	10 mg.
Vitamin B₆	30 mg.	Vitamin B₆	10 mg.
PABA	75 mg.	PABA	25 mg.
Vitamin C	600 mg.	Vitamin C	200 mg.
Vitamin D	2,400 I.U.	Vitamin D	800 I.U.
Potassium	750 mg.	Potassium	250 mg.
Magnesium	300 mg.	Magnesium	100 mg.
Copper	0.6 mg.	Copper	0.2 mg.
Iron	150 mg.	Iron	50 mg.
(ferrous sulfate or gluconate)			
Manganese	30 mg.	Manganese	10 mg.

In metropolitan areas where there are health- or natural-food stores, one should have little difficulty in obtaining the vitamins and minerals in the quantities listed. Slight variations in amounts may be encountered, but if any single item falls within 10 per-cent of the amount recommended, it will work satisfactorily. However, there are millions of people who have never heard of, much less had access to, the various items in the above formulas. I found this out quickly when my book *Nutrition and Your Mind* came out, and I received an avalanche of mail asking me where these formulas were available. My hope is to avoid this

BASIC FAST OXIDIZER SUPPLEMENT

Total Daily Amount		*Each Capsule to Contain*	
Vitamin A	30,000 I.U.	Vitamin A	10,000 I.U.
(*This* **must** be *pal-mitate*, **not** *fish liver oil*)			
Vitamin E	600 I.U.	Vitamin E	200 I.U.
(*This* **must** be "*mixed tocopher-ols*," **not** *Vitamin E acetate*)			
Niacinamide	600 mg.	Niacinamide	200 mg.
Vitamin C	150 mg.	Vitamin C	50 mg.
Choline	600 mg.	Choline	200 mg.
Inositol	150 mg.	Inositol	50 mg.
Calcium	600 mg.	Calcium	200 mg.
Phosphate	600 mg.	Phosphate	200 mg.
Iodine	.045 mg.	Iodine	.015 mg.
Zinc sulfate, oxide, or gluconate	30 mg.	Zinc	10 mg.
Vitamin B$_{12}$	150 mcg.	Vitamin B$_{12}$	50 mcg.

difficulty again, so I have arranged with a wholesale producer*
to make the formulas available at the lowest possible cost.

The following chapter will present several case histories which
illustrate in detail how to control and improve nutrition. Every
book on nutrition I have ever seen treats all persons as though
each had identical needs, and this is *false and misleading,* if one
desires to maximize one's personal strength.

---

* Write to Edom Laboratories, Inc., 860 Grand Blvd., Deer Park, N.Y. 11729. Phone
(516) 586-2266.

5

How to Increase Your
Personality Strength

The psychochemical type one most frequently encounters among those who aren't functioning at their full potential are fast oxidizers. Here is a list of the personality traits most often observed among individuals in this group:

Low self-esteem
("I generally mess things up and always look like a wreck.")

Self-pity
("I asked my mom 'why was I born' and she said she wished she knew. No matter how sick, how tired, how loused up I am, nobody cares at all.")

Pessimism
("Nothing good ever happens to me; I'm getting to the point where I don't give a damn about anything—it's all so depressing.")

Hostility
("Just about everyone I know drives me up the wall. The girls I work with think I like them; well, I'd like them to drop dead.")

Envy
("Her husband buys her anything she wants. They go everywhere. I don't get it—my husband has two college degrees and is ten times smarter than hers.")

66

Anxiety
("I hate this job and everything about the whole place, but I'm afraid all the time; every payday I wake up and say to myself, 'This is it, I'm going to get fired tonight.'")

Lack of ambition, drive
("I can't think of anything I want to do. If I didn't have to work I'd just stay home, take naps, and watch TV.")

Emotional overreaction to everyday difficulties
("When my boss is out of the office and I have to take some of his calls, I'm a three-martini wreck when five o'clock finally rolls around.")

In interviewing and testing volunteer research patients who exhibit these kinds of personality traits one is impressed by the fact that they all consider themselves to be "normal." Their typical reply to questions about how they regard themselves is "I'm okay. Just normal—average, I guess—like my friends."

The following case history illustrates just such a self-styled "normal" person, and also shows how different his *potential* self was from what he had all along thought to be his "normal" self.

One afternoon I met this typically "average" young man, who, as it turned out, exhibited virtually all of the negative personality traits I have just listed.

I was in a foreign car specialist's shop, waiting to have two handmade parts installed in an exotic car on loan from a close friend who was spending a few months in Europe.

I got into a conversation with the machinist who made the parts—a "precision grinder," as he referred to himself. I remarked to him that he must derive considerable satisfaction from his skill at making unobtainable parts for vintage foreign cars.

"I hate it," he said simply, and made a gesture at kicking his lathe. "In fact," he continued, "I hate this whole damned place, and particularly . . ." and here he jerked his head toward an older man who was supervising the work on the car.

Always on the lookout for research patients, I sensed the possibility that here might be a likely candidate, for his negative and hostile remarks might be psychochemical in origin, rather than "normal" psychological reactions to an unfavorable job situation.

I had a long wait for the car—it was promised at one and I drove out at three—so consequently I had a fair chance to become a little acquainted with Jack Young, the angry precision grinder.

After describing the kind of work I did, I gradually eased the conversation around until he became interested, to the point of accepting my invitation to come over and let us run some tests on him. After all, they were free, and they just might lead to something. His knees and feet hurt him, and he said that he "sure would like some 'pep.'"

Here is what he told me about himself in our initial interview:

I was raised by a dominating uncle from about when I was ten years old until I left home at eighteen. He was always critical of everything that I did; always on my back—fourteen hours a day. I finally got up enough nerve to get away, and I joined the Navy, where I was for seven years until I washed out as an aviation cadet. I got along okay in the Navy because no one was after me all the time. The petty officers were on our side, and even though I flunked out, during those seven years I had learned to become a master machinist. That's how I got this job. The boss is killing me but I'm afraid to quit 'cause jobs are hard to find. I get gassed up every weekend so I can forget that I have to go back to that damned job Monday.

Both the blood tests and the Psychochemical Odor Test placed him in the fast oxidizer class. His initial scores on the odor test were 68 on the fast scale and 32 on the slow scale, giving him a score of 28 fast.

Psychochemically this is a *high* score, and is fairly typical of those who exhibit five or more of the psychological traits listed above. Jack "hated his job"—but, he shrugged, "who didn't?" He said he "was no different from anyone else; everyone has these same problems. We're all just human, that's all."

Well, to be sure these are "human difficulties," but they aren't *necessary* ones. They are typical of people who aren't functioning at a normal—much less optimal—biochemical level. There are many possible reasons for this, but suboptimal nutrition is one of the most frequent.

My research interest in Jack Young was to see whether, and if so, how much, we could change his attitudes toward himself, his boss, and his job by improving his biological functioning through orthonutrition.

I began working with him in our standard way: blood tests, psychological assessment on a standard test,° an odor test kit, and a bottle of placebos. He was asked to start the day (before breakfast) by taking and recording his odor test results, together with comments on yesterday's food intake and how he felt at the time he took the odor test. I requested that he mail to me his records for each week (this to help keep him motivated). In addition, he was to take one capsule after each meal. I told him the capsules contained essential vitamins, which they did, but in such minute quantities as to be of no value—for example, one microgram of vitamin B_1.

°The Minnesota Multiphasic Personality Inventory.

Here is his first seven-day set of odor scores, with his comments about how he felt at the time:

	Fast	Slow	Comment
Monday	64	28	—
Tuesday	72	24	"Very depressed"
Wednesday	72	24	"Very depressed"
Thursday	60	36	"Better today— big steak dinner last night"
Friday	72	24	"Way down"
Saturday	64	34	"Picking up"
Sunday	56	40	"Best I've felt in weeks"

These scores average to 35 points fast—worse than when he was first tested (his score then was 28 fast). However, his score on Sunday was down to 16 fast, and he noted that he felt the best he had in weeks. Of course he had been away from his job for two whole days, probably had got "gassed up" (as he called it), and ate better than during the days when he was at work.

Jack was kept on placebos and given no dietary advice for two months. He had been instructed at the beginning not to make any changes whatever in his normal eating and living patterns until we could assess the effect of the pills (placebos).

The following quotations, taken from his medical records, tell what happened when we switched him from placebos to the rather potent nutritional supplement, and gave him the diet for fast oxidizers, which included the optimum amount of protein for his weight:

After two months on placebos: "I feel about the same. I'm unhappy with that job and I hate the boss more every week."

After two months of orthonutrition: "I'm getting along pretty good at work. Things don't seem to bother me so much. I'm eating regularly like you told me to. I guess you could say that I just feel better generally."

After five months' orthonutrition: "I'm a lot more peppy. Sharp all around. [An impudent grin.] I don't mind telling anybody anything. My optimism is pretty high, and I don't worry about anything at work anymore. It's hard for me to remember why I used to feel sorry for myself."

At the start of Jack's placebo trial his average score for a week on the Psychochemical Odor Test was 35 points fast. At his worst, at the end of one week on placebos, he had an average score of 35 points fast, and on three days he had reported scores of 48 fast—the maximum the test records. His score on the day he made the preceding remarks was *2 points slow.*

After six months' orthonutrition: "Great. I'm thinking a lot about the future. I just got the idea that I don't *have* to be a precision grinder for the rest of my life. My brother works on a tuna boat out of San Pedro. He really likes it."

His odor test score this day was 4 points fast. I might remark here again that scores of 6 points fast or slow are normal. In fact, some people are most highly motivated when their scores are from 2 to 4 points slow; it's an individual matter, however.

After nine months' orthonutrition: "Really okay. I'm pepped up a lot. I don't worry about anything. I got fired from my job Friday for sassing my boss. To hell with 'em; I don't give a damn. I'll do something *I* want to do."

After one year of orthonutrition: "Went to the bank with my brother and borrowed money to buy a fishing boat from the guy my brother's been working for. He's old and wants to take it easy. I feel great all around."

After eighteen months on the orthonutritional program: "Now fishing for a living. Boy, a lot has happened to me since I met you. It's great!"

It required from three to five months on the ortho diet and supplements for Jack's "personality" to begin to show a sharp shift toward normality. During this period his average scores on the Psychochemical Odor Test were 4 points fast/slow (plus or minus 2). No changes had to be made in his basic nutritional supplement, which is unusual. The psychological summary in his chart reads: (1) self-esteem up; (2) self-pity gone; (3) pessimism gone; (4) hostility redirected to normal aggressiveness; (5) anxiety gone; (6) ambition way up—completely redirected his lifestyle; (7) now able to shrug off normal everyday vexations.

To someone who has never witnessed such a personality reconstruction, the case of Jack Young might seem unusual, if not impossible. However, it is neither unusual nor impossible. It is what I expect, and what I find, in case after case after case, in those persons who are found to be not functioning at their optimum biochemical levels. And, as I have said, more than psychological evaluation or biochemical indices, the Psychochemical Odor Test is always our single most valuable index. It is not only the most sensitive, but it is the only test which *zeroes in on the individual*. You do it *yourself;* you do not require the analysis and advice of anyone because the test tells you something you need to know about yourself—that no one else knows. And, perhaps most important, you know this fundamentally crucial information *when you need to know it.* No blood tests or tests of any other kind deliver a virtually instant insight into what is going on in your tissues as they turn food into energy.

The following are some further case histories of changes in lifestyle in persons using the Psychochemical Odor Test as a guide to orthonutrition.

Harold Parks, a former student and research patient of mine, initially described himself as a "neurotic mess." After treatment, he embarked on a successful career as an advertising salesman. When he called me to say he was in town and just wanted to say "hello," I invited him to come to dinner. In accepting the invitation he asked if he could bring a friend—someone who might be of interest to me. She was a young woman who was a graduate student at a nearby university.

We spent a pleasant social evening together, but my professional interests kept intruding because I was both intrigued and puzzled by the young woman.

I'll call her Cathy. She said she was twenty-five, had a degree in social studies, and was now working on a research project which sort of combined environmental concerns with sociology. If this sounds vague and makes you wonder, it sounded just that way to me.

I tried to get her to tell me just exactly what she was doing, what kind of data she was collecting, what the aim of the study was, etc. But she was simply vague—even vacuous—about the whole thing. Although she said she was twenty-five, her voice pattern and general social demeanor were those of about a fifteen-year-old. She was hesitant in speech, shy, and appeared to be sort of lost in a world that was far too much for her.

The next day Harold phoned me.

"What did you think of Cathy?" he asked.

I told him that I could hardly believe she was twenty-five years old. She both acted and appeared to be in her middle teens.

"Exactly," he replied. "She is the daughter of a physician, a very good friend of mine, and I've wanted you to get a look at her for a long time. Last night was my chance."

Of course I was interested immediately in enlisting her as a research patient, and asked him to have her call me for an appointment.

"No way. Absolutely," was his answer. "You scared the hell out of her. She said you were mean and overbearing. She won't have anything to do with you at all."

I asked him if *he* thought I had been mean and overbearing

toward her, and he said, "Absolutely not. Cathy reacts that way to a lot of people. I know she's had a lot of psychological counseling. Also, she says funny things like 'I don't know who I am.' She also cries easily and a lot."

I asked him if he still had the odor kit I had given him. He said he had it, but seldom used it since "he had gotten himself pretty well together. I only use it if I'm slumping or something."

I then asked if there were any way he could persuade Cathy to record odor responses before breakfast for a week or two, keeping any reference to me out of it. She certainly knew he had been a patient of mine. If she admitted having any emotional difficulties, she might also welcome help from a friend. Harold said he thought he could get her to use the odor test.

My plan was to get the odor reports from Harold, and then tell him what he should advise her to do. I hoped to improve Cathy's biological functioning to the point where she might not be so meek and frightened, and might even consent to make an appointment to come and see me. About a month later the mail brought eight little slips of paper with odor test scores written on them, together with a note from Harold explaining that this was the best he could do. The test dates were not consecutive, he said, because Cathy wasn't interested enough to use the test. Here are the scores that she recorded:

Date	Fast Oxidizer	Slow Oxidizer
1/12	32	64
1/13	28	64
1/20	24	72
1/21	24	72
1/29	36	60
2/4	40	56
2/5	32	64
2/6	28	64

These average out to about 30 on the fast scale and 64 on the slow scale—a 34-point difference. Briefly, then, her score was 34 slow. This is almost exactly the score Jack Young, the precision grinder, recorded at the start of his program, but his score was on the fast, not the slow side.

I was not surprised by Cathy's high score, but I was considerably surprised to discover that Cathy appeared to be a slow oxidizer. (Only a very small percentage—less than ten—of our female research patients have been slow oxidizers. I don't know why.)

In a way I was relieved. Slow oxidizing is generally easier to correct, and the results of treatment are more impressive. Since Harold had been a slow oxidizer, things appeared to be quite simple.

I sent Harold a brief note asking him to try to get Cathy to follow the same general diet and take the same vitamin-mineral supplements that he had started on. A week or so later I received a reply saying that Cathy agreed to follow the diet and take supplements. "Good news," I thought, and wondered how long it would take for Cathy to respond to her orthonutritional program: certainly not more than a month or two.

When it is said that about 90 percent of the energy produced by the brain is derived from blood sugar, what is really meant is that this energy is derived from glucose *and* oxygen:

glucose + oxygen = energy + carbon dioxide + water

One important aspect of the body's use of oxygen is that it does not seem to be able to take in more than is required for immediate use. For example, the body at rest consumes about 0.21 liters per minute; walking rapidly, 2.5 liters per minute; running, 3.0 liters per minute.

The capacity of the blood for transporting oxygen is determined by the amount of the carrying agent *hemoglobin* present in the bloodstream. For adult males this ranges from 13.5 to 18.0 grams per 100 milliliters of blood; in adult females the normal range is from 11.5 to 16.4 grams per 100 milliliters of blood.

Many factors affect these levels: vitamins and minerals (principally iron, vitamin B_{12}, folic acid, vitamin C) as well as other nutrients such as protein and essential fatty acids. The final, and for some persons *most important*, factor is physical exercise. Given all the essential nutritional factors, one can *increase* one's utilization of oxygen by increasing the body's need for it. In other words, a slow oxidizer can increase his or her oxidation rate by exercise.

Considerations such as these made me uneasy about Cathy: I had no blood tests on her. When I asked Harold if he had any idea when she last had had a physical examination, he said he knew that a physical was required of all newly entering women students at the university. But this didn't answer the questions I wanted answers to. All it meant to me was that she was well enough to go to school. So when I heard nothing from either of them for over two months I began to wonder.

I didn't have much longer to speculate, however, for about seven o'clock one evening I received a telephone call from Cathy. Her voice was barely audible; also, she sounded as if she was trying to talk while crying. She told me she was very depressed and needed help and reassurance.

I immediately wanted to know if she still had the odor kit, and if so, would she get it and tell me on the phone what her responses to the six vials were on the fast and slow oxidizer scales. She said she had the kit, she got it, and reported that all six odors on the slow oxidizing scale smelled like "burning trash"—meaning her score was the maximum the test recorded for a slow oxidizer. She said she was just getting over the flu—doubtless a contributing factor—but she said she really hadn't felt much better on the orthonutritional program; "perhaps a little," she said.

I told her to drink two large glasses of orange juice immediately, take a double dose of the vitamin-mineral formula for slow oxidizers, go for a brisk walk for about thirty minutes, and call me back after she had rested about twenty minutes after the walk.

An hour later she called and said she was feeling much better and "would be okay." Her voice was much stronger and she said how grateful she was for my fast and sympathetic aid.

The slow oxidizer, you will recall, is not turning blood sugar into energy at a normal rate. This has a particularly adverse effect upon psychological functions, since the nervous system is almost totally dependent upon blood sugar for its proper functioning. And the nervous system includes the brain. Many other factors are involved in these metabolic processes as well. Hormones, vitamins, minerals, foods other than carbohydrates, and so on are necessary for building red blood cells. One of these factors is often overlooked because it is so familiar: one's *oxygen consumption* is of critical importance.

When Cathy told me she hadn't improved significantly on the slow oxidizer diet and nutritional supplements, I immediately suspected a possible deficiency in the oxygen-carrying capacity of her blood. I had been through this before with other patients whose blood hemoglobin was "low normal," and in fact when I finally received a blood count on Cathy her hemoglobin turned out to be only 12—just about the bottom of the so-called normal range.

Since Cathy hadn't improved on the orthodiet, clearly what she was receiving was not complete. The missing factor in her case was indeed exercise, or more precisely, oxygen consumption. Unless one's blood carries an optimum amount, total nutrition *cannot* be achieved. Oxygen is an essential nutrient. I realize that one does not ordinarily think of oxygen or water as "nutrients," but I am using this term to emphasize the importance of aspects of one's nutritional state that are almost universally overlooked when one talks or thinks about nutrition.

With the consent of her physician—an absolute *must* for anyone beginning an exercise program—Cathy enrolled in a physical fitness class at the university, while continuing the orthonutritional program.

I heard no more from or about her for many months, until her friend Harold called one morning and asked me and my wife to dinner, saying he had a surprise for us. We were to meet at a restaurant at eight—a meeting I'm not likely ever to forget.

He appeared with a young woman whose name was Cathy. This was the name of the girl that I had met over a year ago— when she appeared to be a withdrawn, immature teenager. Now I was confronted with a mature, poised, handsome young woman who simply bore no resemblance at all to the Cathy I had first met. She was smiling, friendly, talked freely and confidently, and had changed physically from a frail little girl into a very confident, intelligent, attractive adult. Gone were the vague, overly idealistic notions about saving the world; she was on her way to law school; her goal: to become a corporation lawyer.

She told me that she was running a mile every other day; her hemoglobin was averaging around 15.5; and her score on the Psychochemical Odor Test generally was between 2 and 4 slow.

Several years later I met her at a social gathering. She had finished law school and was now employed by one of the big law firms that handled the legal affairs of several large (worldwide) corporations. Her goal? She sort of half laughed when she said it, but she wanted to become one of the first women lawyers to become a partner in the firm.

Exceptional? Yes, by ordinary current establishment psychological theories of motivation. But definitely not when judged by the personality changes and hence in the lifestyles of those who have participated in the orthonutritional program.

Assuming that the latent genetic ability is there, and that the biochemical potential is being fulfilled by an optimum and correct orthonutritional program, then the maximum personality strength of the individual can be realized. Cathy apparently had the correct genes—lawyers ran in the family—and the orthodietary program allowed her latent hereditary endowment to be expressed.

However, the latent hereditary endowment—the full personality potential—is not always all that one would wish. The following case history is an illustration.

Joe was a two-hundred-pound, tall, muscular twenty-year-old with a luxuriant black beard. He appeared to be a gentle person, soft-spoken and unusually polite (he rose if I got up and remained standing until I sat down).

He was referred to us by a social worker, a woman whose son had benefited from participating in our program. Here is what she told me about Joe:

"He has had several minor brushes with the law, twice for 'joyriding' (appropriating an unlocked car, cruising around for a few hours, and then abandoning the car); twice for illegal possession of liquor (beer and whiskey); once for disorderly conduct (participating in a street fight).

"None of this is really serious or too unusual for a big, strong young man who has too much time on his hands. What I think he needs is the kind of biochemical lift you gave my son, so that he can set some goals and get going on a creative path."

At the time, Joe had a juvenile court record and was on probation. His coming to see me was not voluntary. The social worker was his probation officer.

This kind of setup was not to my liking; I didn't think he would really cooperate under legal duress. Consequently, I decided not to treat him as a research patient (no placebos), but just try to optimize his nutrition by having him come to see me weekly so that I could check his progress, if any.

We found his blood tests to be normal; he also scored zero (48 fast/48 slow) on the Psychochemical Odor Test. Since he was neither a fast nor a slow oxidizer, the only possibility left was that he might be a suboxidizer—which seemed extremely unlikely to me. He was simply a big, strong, healthy young man. But I had agreed to put him into our program, and I kept my promise because on his psychological test he registered a rather high score on the scale which measures social conformity: he most certainly was a nonconformer—but sometimes such nonconformity is really hostility. If such was the case with Joe, then there might be a chance that we could redirect this general hostility into goal-directed ambition of a socially constructive kind.

But I wouldn't have wagered a postage stamp on it.

Consequently I gave him the dietary instructions for suboxidizers, plus the rather potent vitamin-mineral supplement that was to be taken with the diet. I made an appointment for him to return for an appraisal in about ten days.

He didn't return. Instead, about two months later I received a call from the social worker telling me that Joe "had a little more trouble." His father owned a rather large salvage company. Joe worked for him and was caught stealing a truckload of valuable salvage (automobile engines and transmissions). He was selling them through an intermediary to some of his father's competitors—one of whom recognized a certain engine and transmission and told Joe's father he ought to make a careful check of his inventory. The father acted immediately. He knew the thief could only have been the one person who had access to the stolen goods, his son Joe.

The father called the social worker, asking that this not be reported to the juvenile authorities. He wanted it kept a "family affair." The social worker agreed, saying that, since Joe was under treatment, a little patience might resolve the problem.

Consequently Joe returned to see me. Now, however, he was not quite the gentle, soft-spoken person I had first met a little over two months before.

His response to my usual first question about how he had been getting along drew this response: "I've felt better, really better. In fact I don't ever remember feeling so good. I've got real energy—I sometimes keep going all day and night just for the hell of it."

When asked what he did at such times, he said, "Oh, just cruise around, looking for action."

Well, action was what he soon got. About three weeks after this conversation I received a telephone call from the social worker, who told me that the day before at about three A.M., he was seen by officers in a cruising police car as he was trying to pry open a first-floor window at the rear of Juvenile Hall. Joe spotted the police car, which was going down a side street past the alley behind Juvenile Hall. Joe had had the foresight to park his car in the alley approximately in front of the window he was trying to open. The police car was proceeding in a direction which was at a right angle to the alley, so they were going away from where Joe emerged from the alley.

"Joe shot out of the alley, made a sharp right turn, and raced down the street to a rather narrow two-lane highway which led into the country. By this time the police were in a daring competition with a nut who was driving a 'muscle' car that had more power than any police car.

"The police radioed ahead for help to cut Joe off at a junction about five miles out of town. They were moving at speeds up to 145 mph, but the added police reinforcements met Joe at the intersection and forced him off the road into a field, where his car overturned and caught fire.

"One police car which tried to force him off the road was sideswiped; two officers were injured."

I asked her how she possessed such detailed information of the incident, and she said she was at police headquarters and was reading from the official police report, adding a few details of her own that she had obtained from Joe, who was unhurt and in jail.

The social worker later told me that Joe was trying to get into Juvenile Hall to steal the file they had on him. He had "cased the joint" (his language) and knew just where his file was kept. She also told me that the police report said that at the time of arrest "the suspect showed no evidence of being under the influence of either alcohol or drugs."

I asked her if Joe showed any signs of remorse or regret when she interviewed him the day of his arrest. Her answer didn't surprise me.

She said, "Hardly. He was elated, excited, and high; and told me he had never before realized what a 'thrill' was."

This whole episode and the events leading into it provide a good example of the kind of person we call a "psychopath."

The dramatic change in Joe's personality from general mild passivity—soft-spoken, unusually polite gentleness—to daring criminal behavior "just for the hell of it" can only be attributed to the biochemical changes in him resulting from the realization of his full personality potential: the result of the orthonutritional program he was following. After he had been in jail a short time awaiting trial, his social worker said he withdrew into his "former self." Clearly, jail food does not constitute orthonutrition.

Joe unfortunately stumbled into an opportunity for realizing his full personality potential, just as did Cathy. But one became a felon, while the other became a successful lawyer.

I wish I could say that Joe represents a rare, isolated case. Although negative changes in lifestyle are not common, I can cite many others. Here are three:

A sixteen-year-old male who cornered both parents in the kitchen, waving a butcher knife at them (a younger sister called the police).

A thirty-year-old male who admitted he deliberately led a motorcycle officer on a speed chase so that he could jump him and beat him up when the officer "caught" him.

A twenty-five-year-old woman who smashed all the furniture in her room and critically injured her father by hitting him with a bronze lamp when he tried to interfere.

Each of these cases had been referred to us by friends who had previously participated in the orthonutrition program. And each had volunteered to become a research patient because they said they were "tired all the time," "lacked ambition," "couldn't stick to anything," and so on.

Biochemically they all were classified as suboxidizers, which indeed proved to be correct, since when they were put on the ortho program for suboxidizers their latent abilities to produce energy became all too evident.

Although one rarely encounters this type of research patient, I have since learned to introduce and gradually increase segments of the program bit by bit while keeping a close lookout for early indications of energy surges and the channels they might lead into. The Minnesota Multiphasic Personality Inventory is a sensitive test which reveals changes in areas that might be undesirable (I direct this last comment to psychotherapists).

For the average person using the Psychochemical Odor Test as a guide to improved psychological and emotional performance only one thing must be kept in mind. If, after being on the full program for a month or two, one finds oneself hyperactive, taking on too much and overdoing it all the way round, the amount of the nutritional supplement should be gradually decreased until this accelerated emotional and psychological state subsides. (It will, and very quickly too—say, a few days—because, as soon as your tissues no longer have access to the energy-producing substances you have been giving them daily, they cannot function at full capacity.) The negative changes in behavior (mentioned above) have principally involved males. However, one hardly expects females not to react similarly negatively and in the same proportions to the general population as do males. Here is an interesting and unusual case history:

Barbara B. was the twenty-three-year-old daughter of parents long prominent in motion pictures and in television. She was born and raised in the privileged community of the rich and famous clustered around Beverly Hills. Her mother described her to me as attractive, well educated, talented, chic, and socially poised. Her parents were concerned because, as they put it, "she won't *do anything*." They felt that there must be something physically wrong with her because her don't-give-a-damn attitude emerged gradually after she finished college. Her mother also said that after almost two years of psychoanalysis her daughter had not changed at all.

Barbara B. had experienced a brief period of rebellion as a college sophomore—smoked some marijuana, wore some "far-out" clothes—but, according to her mother, this period lasted only a year or so.

Barbara B. agreed to come to see me through the influence of a friend, a young man whom I had known socially for many years. It is of some clinical interest to know that she would not come to her appointment alone, but was brought to the interview by her friend, and she wanted him to be present during our interview. She was timid, all right, one would almost say frightened, not of me particularly, but of any new situation.

Of the eight most frequently observed kinds of personality traits mentioned above (pages 66–67), she checked the following five on a brief personality quiz:

1. *Low self-esteem.*
2. *Continuous, mild background depression.*
3. *Anxiety.*
4. *Lack of energy/low level of interest.*
5. *Emotional overreaction to everyday difficulties.*

We classified her as a fast oxidizer on the bases of her blood tests and the Psychochemical Odor Test. On the latter her scores were fast 60, slow 44, for a net score of 16 fast.

The diet survey she completed revealed that she practically lived on the very foods fast oxidizers are asked to avoid:

Typical breakfast:
Black coffee, pastry, glass of skim milk.

Typical lunch:
Cottage cheese and lettuce salad, with soda crackers and a dietary cola drink.

Typical dinner:
Small serving of chicken or fish, potatoes, salad, pie or cake, black coffee.

In sum, a high-starch-sugar, low-protein, low-vitamin-mineral diet.

She said she was about ten pounds underweight, but couldn't gain because she wasn't interested in food: "I'm just never hungry." This is a typical response for fast oxidizers. With test scores such as Barbara's, one suspects the beginning of anorexia nervosa (nervous loss of appetite). The remedy here is to change the food-intake pattern entirely (to foods recommended for fast oxidizers; she was eating mainly items recommended for slow ozidizers). This dietary change will bring the biochemical balance back to normal—Psychochemical Odor Test score around 4 points either fast or slow—and with this change the appetite returns. Needless to say, it is often very difficult to get people to do this, because of long-standing habits. But it can be done.

The Psychochemical Odor Test provided the stimulus to get Barbara to agree to try to change her diet. She had majored in psychology in college, and had never heard of—and didn't believe in—the possibility that the sense of smell could be *altered* by what one did or didn't eat.

I didn't attempt to argue the point. I just asked her to take an odor kit home with her, change her diet according to the instructions given in the Psychochemical Odor Test manual, take the vitamin-mineral supplements as indicated by her scores on the test, and keep a daily record of these scores together with what she had eaten that day.

A month later, at about the time I had scheduled a second appointment for her, I received a telephone call from her mother asking me to *send* a new supply of the vitamin-mineral supplement for her daughter. Or, if it would be more convenient for me, her mother said she would send her car and driver over to pick them up.

I had never faced this kind of request before, and I was a bit irritated by the subtle commanding attitude behind it (I have long since learned to avoid wealthy, prominent types; they are impossible research patients). When I asked Barbara's mother why her daughter couldn't keep her appointment, I received the surprising answer; "Barbara's too busy right now to spend the better part of an afternoon coming all the way from Beverly Hills to your office."

I learned that Barbara's business was purely social. She had a house guest, a former college roommate, and they were looking up old friends and having social gatherings.

Since these activities meant that Barbara had suddenly come to life, I agreed to send the vitamin-mineral formula if Barbara would do two things: mail me her odor test scores and agree to keep an appointment with me about a month later. I added that I would send the nutritional supplements as soon as I received the odor test records from her. By this arrangement I would have information I needed about the biochemical state of the patient before continuing the treatment.

A few days later I actually received Barbara's odor test scores covering about a three-week period (several days were missing; "I was not home," she wrote). In an accompanying letter she said she was following the program faithfully and was feeling much, much better. She apologized for missing her appointment, but assured me she would see me on time next month.

When I had run the Psychochemical Odor Test on her during our initial interview her score was 16 fast. The test results she recorded at home showed that in a little over two weeks her score had shifted from fast to normal, and was at last reading 2 points slow. For most people their energy is highest when the score is a little on the slow side, say, up to 4 or 5 points. Individuals differ on this matter, as would be expected. But anyone using the test regularly can soon establish the test score at which he or she feels strongest: highest motivation, more confidence, more achievement. Barbara's social re-emergence fits into the pattern of being at her best when her score is a little on the slow side. Her rapid switch in biochemical balance was not unusual for a young, healthy woman who only required a push in the right direction in order to get her going.

Consequently I sent a month's supply of the nutritional supplement with a note suggesting she continue the diet but also watch her odor test score; it ought not to get slower than 6.

In some persons, when the oxidation rate as indicated on the Psychochemical Odor Test gets a little too slow—say, 8 to 10 points—they become overaggressive, irritable, and easily affronted. And once in a while they may do impulsive, strange things that they normally would never think of doing. I didn't know Barbara well enough to know whether she might fit into this group. But I was not thinking of these possibilities when I sent Barbara her vitamin-mineral supplement, principally because the point is covered in the odor test manual I gave her to use as a guide.

Barbara kept her next appointment as promised. Her appearance, however, had changed. When I first interviewed her she wore a tailored light blue pants suit with darker blue shoes and carried a matching blue handbag. I noted this on her chart because her costume was so different from what I was accustomed to seeing on young women (Levi's and T-shirts) that I considered her conservative dress might have clinical significance. Now her feet were bare in leather sandals, her dress was something filmy, long, and flowing, reminding one of India, and she wore several strands of multicolored, waist-length beads. I supposed it to be most likely that her new costume reflected her new contacts with old friends.

Psychologically she was about what I expected: she was cheerful, outgoing, and relaxed; and she came alone and had driven herself from Beverly Hills to Pasadena. "It's real fun to be driving again. I stopped about two years ago—I was too afraid."

I showed her the psychological quiz she had checked at our first interview: low self-esteem, depression, anxiety, low energy, and emotional overreaction to everyday difficulties. She glanced at the list and said, "There really have been some definite changes that I like, but I seem to be getting more intolerant. You know, my parents are laying it on me pretty heavy. They're just not with it."

I should have caught the possible significance of this last remark. But I was so pleased with her improvement generally that I saw no reason to modify or change the direction of her treatment. However, I really slipped up when she scored 8 slow on the Psychochemical Odor Test, for this *could* mean trouble—and I missed it.

She agreed to come back in a month for a re-evaluation of the nutritional program she was following; but I never saw her again. I telephoned her home twice and was told she was not there. I left messages both times to have her call me. She didn't.

After three months had passed I got in touch with the friend who had brought her to her first interview. He sort of laconically said, "Barbara? Oh, she's dropped out. She's into the drug scene on the strip."°

I have been citing case histories of changes in lifestyles which have occurred when an individual's total personality strength is realized by orthonutritional treatment. Achieving "total personality strength" (or something close to it) sometimes entails achieving "total disaster."

I have never attempted a systematic study of the differences between men and women in the directions negative personality changes take, principally because of the sheer magnitude of the task. Only one negative change in lifestyle occurs to approximately four hundred positive changes. In order to have a research group of thirty negatives (the minimum), one would have

---

° The strip is a section of Sunset Boulevard, between Hollywood and Beverly Hills, where pimps, prostitutes, drug users, and drug pushers hang out.

to have a total number of research subjects of many thousands. Further, this number would have to be *doubled* to compare men and women. So let's just forget it.

However, on the basis of the limited data that I *do* have— *which by no means can be considered scientific evidence*—the negative lifestyles that have emerged in our male research subjects have all been toward violence and actual criminal behavior, while the negative changes in lifestyle of the women have all been toward self-destruction (alcohol, narcotics) and sexual promiscuity (including prostitution).

The following is a typical example of the kind of negative lifestyle that emerges in women. A quite plain eighteen-year-old who "had never had a date," was "always into a book," began first to lose her interest in books, then joined a young people's church group, where she met a compatible man, switched from him to another, and a year later (she told me) was occasionally being picked up by a stranger in a singles bar; one of these strangers introduced her to drugs.

While I could cite many other similar examples, it would be simply boring, for they all exhibit the following general pattern: from lack of interest in men and sexual ignorance and passivity, to sort of "suddenly" discovering men as objects of interest, to initially subtle advances leading to a first success in attracting a man, then attracting others, and others, and so on.

Where all this leads I do not know, because once their energy level rises and their full personality potential begins to set goals and shape behavior, I rarely ever see them again.

6

Sex and Personality

One inevitably encounters sex as an aspect of personality when doing the kind of research reported in this book—studies broadly directed at discovering connections between body chemistry and thought, feeling, and behavior. I make this comment only to emphasize that, even though sexual behavior may not be a primary research target, the subject emerges when one induces personality changes in research patients by increasing (or inadvertently decreasing) their levels of energy production.

My first encounter with the possibility of a *direct* connection between sex drive and nutritional biochemistry was an eye-opener for me and a brief disaster for the victim.

In connection with a campaign they were planning for a pharmaceutical company for which I was a consultant, two aggressive advertising men interviewed me several times. One day at lunch we were discussing the subject of nutrition and energy. Later, one of the men, Jim, asked me to recommend an all-purpose vitamin-mineral supplement for him, because he said he wanted to "cover all the bases" in keeping his capacity for work high.

At that time I was groping with the problems of biochemical imbalances, and in fact knew very little about what effects a given vitamin-mineral combination might have on the energy-producing systems of the body. I had been taught, as all biochemists seemed to believe, that essential nutrients—up to the maximum an individual could utilize—were beneficial both in promoting tissue repair and in energy production.

What I didn't know—and it took years to find out why—was that this general belief of biochemists is false and that certain vitamins and minerals in selected patients would actually *lower* their energy production.

So in my academic ignorance I gave Jim a standard high-potency all-purpose vitamin-mineral combination and suggested he take six capsules a day. I didn't know then that the combination I gave him would *increase* his oxidation rate; in retrospect, I know that Jim was a fast oxidizer and that what I gave him was about the very last thing he needed.

Three weeks later he phoned me, asking, "What kind of a dirty bastard are you, anyway?" He didn't seem to be joking, either.

He had suddenly become impotent—and just at the beginning of an affair he had been working for a long time to set up. He blamed my pills for his impotence, for he said, "Nothing like this has ever happened to me before. Hell," he went on, "I'm a *tiger* in bed, and now look what you've done to me."

His friend, the other advertising man, later told me that he also thought that I had deliberately slipped the sex knockout pills to Jim as a practical joke.

I am not a practical joker nor was I at all convinced that the vitamin-mineral formula I gave Jim had anything to do with his sudden impotence. But *he* believed it, and said that a few days after stopping the pills he was back to his former vigor.

Since I was completely unconvinced that the nutritional supplements I gave Jim were connected with his episode of impotence—it lasted about ten days—I wanted more information. So I explained to Jim that there was some kind of a mixup in the lab, obviously, otherwise this couldn't have happened. I told him I would check, and if a mistake had been made it could be corrected. I would give him the correct formula, which not only could sustain his sex drive, but maintain it at a high level. At any rate, I said, it's worth a try. He agreed.

For research purposes we had experimental formulas made up in batches of ten thousand capsules, and we varied the colors of the capsules from batch to batch, such as brown/yellow, blue/white, red/white, as well as clear gelatin capsules. The contents of the different-colored capsules were identical. But we used the different colors as a precaution against a patient's possible suggestibility—an additional way to check the "placebo effect."

A few days later Jim stopped by my office and I gave him a supply of the "new" capsules. His original supply had been brown and yellow; these were bright red and white. Their contents, however, were identical.

He was a little down that day, saying he could "really use a boost in energy."

Quite a long time passed and I had no word from him, until I ran into him by chance. He was with several others, entering a restaurant just as I was leaving. He excused himself from his group to speak briefly with me on a social level. As we parted he said, "By the way, I've decided I definitely don't need *any kind* of vitamins."

The brief hint I received from this episode alerted me to include questions concerning one's level of sex interest and activity on the psychological quiz that new research patients were asked to answer.

When one considers that our research patients were all volunteers, seeking help for what they considered to be physical deficiencies of one kind or another, one might expect to find low or nonexistent levels of interest in either the subject of sex or in sexual activity itself. And this is what we have in fact found. This is not surprising, since "fatigue" was the most frequently encountered complaint.

However, such a finding as this means little in itself. It only raises the question of whether or not such lack of interest in sex—including impotence or frigidity—is related to one's *general* level of biochemical energy production. In other words, when a patient's personality strength is increased, is this generally accompanied by renewed or increased interest in sex?

Before reviewing several case histories which may suggest answers to this question, let us consider one of the principal difficulties one must keep in mind when discussing sexual attitudes and behavior.

Sexual inhibition is taught at a very early age, and the teaching continues well into adolescence. It may be that young people who have strong or potentially strong personalities absorb antisexual indoctrination more completely than their weaker peers. This complicates scientific assessment.

Some research patients who show marked improvements in personality strength can also show decreased interest in sex. The treatment releases their potential *for inhibition.*

I first encountered this reaction in a young man who was attending a theological seminary. After three months of orthonutritional treatment he told me that not only was he studying longer, concentrating better, and getting better grades, but he was a much more moral person. "My commitment to God has been strengthened; I'm much abler to control 'wayward' [i.e., sexual] fantasies; I'm a much *better person* [i.e., more 'moral,' 'less sinful']—I can cope with temptation."

In the above case, increased psychological and emotional

strength merely strengthened lifetime acquired inhibitions. The reverse possibility is that with a more dynamic, forceful personality one might overcome one's early negative training. This transformation is comparable to what happens in some individuals during adolescence, when glandular activities are at their peak, and sexual prohibitions administered from early childhood into adolescence often dissolve into teenage pregnancies. Her parents tried to teach her not to, but her hormones had the final say.

The following is a case with an unusual aspect:

A thirty-five-year-old social worker, who told me that she was "ground down" by her responsibilities, improved over a three-month period to where she said she was now enjoying her work and was considering continuing her education. She also, for the first time, brought up the subject of sex. "I thought you might be interested in another change in me. I've always been sort of afraid of men, but I like and even love some women. But I don't like myself as a lover of women, and I've always wished I didn't. Now, however, I don't feel that I *have* to. I can go my own way and be like other women who are attracted to men."

Such a shift in orientation may be interpreted in different ways: increased ability to hold back her basic sexual orientation toward women, or an actual change in the direction of that orientation from women to men. Of course, the entire subject of human sexuality is complex and little understood, but the point at which it intersects with nutritional biochemistry is a field of scientific research that should be pursued.

The following is a related case with a reverse twist:

A twenty-two-year-old male college student, who was failing in two out of five courses, told me, "I can't study—no concentration at all. I guess I'm just going to have to drop out." The trouble with this was that he was engaged to be married the following June, after he finished college. He also had a job lined up (his major was business administration). He was at that time about halfway through the fall semester, and I suggested he withdraw from school for medical reasons, to resume when he felt better.

He responded rapidly to being relieved of the pressures of college and being placed on the orthonutritional program. I thought his progress was so great that he might be able to re-enter school for the spring semester, when I received a phone call from him, telling me he was in "real trouble." He had picked up a young male hitchhiker, taken him to a motel, and seduced him.

The hitchhiker reported this to the police, and my patient was arrested. When he came to trial the judge placed him on probation, on the condition that he undergo psychiatric treatment, which he did. He also continued on the orthonutritional program for another six months.

He was able to finish college, but he didn't get married. Now, three years later, he is an active homosexual with a good job and no regrets.

He told me, "I'm glad I found out as soon as I did—before I got married. I like girls, but somehow I've always been uneasy with them. I don't feel this way at all with men."

In addition to the kinds of changes in sexual attitudes and behavior resulting from orthonutritional treatment which the preceding cases illustrate, even cases of frank impotence in men and frigidity in women have responded to the orthonutritional program. For instance, once I received a letter from a former patient, a heavy-construction worker, who had moved to a new area. Here is part of what he wrote:

My doctor tells me that I ought to take at least three months' leave from my job. I'm only 53 years old and I feel like I'm falling apart. I

can't sleep at night—I just lie still with my eyes closed. I'm also impotent. I can't take three months off—I can't afford to. But I can take six
weeks off on my insurance. My doctor says I'm going through the
"male change of life" and I'll just have to adjust to it, for there is nothing he can do for me. You helped me before when I was rundown. Is
there anything you could suggest for me to try now? I'm desperate.

I had not seen this patient for ten years, and he now lived four
hundred miles from my office. The only thing I could do was to
ask him to have his doctor perform our basic blood tests,° while
I sent our Psychochemical Odor Test kit and manual, asking him
to keep daily, before-breakfast reports of his reactions.

In about two weeks I received both the blood test results and
the Psychochemical Odor Test scores. The blood tests placed him
at almost the extreme end of the Slow Oxidizer scale, while the
Psychochemical Odor Tests averaged 40 points slow. Scores such
as this generally spell real trouble; I was consequently not too optimistic about the eventual outcome. However, I sent him the
appropriate orthonutritional supplements and the manual containing the dietary instructions he was to follow.

At the end of the first month's treatment there was only a
slight shift toward increasing his oxygen consumption: an eight-
point improvement from 40 slow to 32 slow. This was hopeful,
but that's about all. His physical condition had not changed; he
was still exhausted, sleepless, and impotent.

Since normally in situations such as this one finds considerable
improvement in a month, I called him on the phone just to question him in detail to make sure he was doing what I had asked
him to.

He was. But he made one remark that caught my attention: "I
lie still all night and sit still all day."

° Complete blood count, thyroid function, fasting blood sugar level, plasma pH, total
carbon dioxide, carbonic acid, total lipids (includes cholesterol and triglycerides).

The missing factor in his treatment might be poor oxygen consumption. I told him to ask his doctor to approve a program of exercise for him. The doctor agreed and suggested "jogging in place," beginning at five minutes a day, working up to around fifteen, or to when he was breathing deeply and sweating lightly.

End of case: back at work in another month; sexual vigor normal at the end of three months. The patient's final comment, in a letter expressing his gratitude: "I never thought I would ever feel this good again."

In general, any wide variation from the normal rate at which one turns food into energy, repairs tissues, and produces hormones will result in loss of libido—loss of sexuality. In cases such as the one we have just considered—a middle-aged man who had done physical work all of his life—it is not surprising that biochemical functioning would decline with increasing age and unremitting daily strenuous work.

Advancing age and simply wearing out are only two of many causes, however, for biochemical imbalances which affect sexuality. Often one discovers such problems in what appear to be unusually strong, young women and men.

Not long ago I was participating in a television talk show which accepted telephone calls from viewers. The subject of sex and personality was briefly touched upon, and I remarked that, in general, the stronger the personality the stronger the sex drive.

I no sooner had made this comment than the interviewer put a call on the line, a young woman, who said flatly that this simply was not true—even in a general sense (allowing an occasional exception). She said that she felt she had a strong personality, but that sex was simply nothing at all for her, and she wondered whether there was something wrong with me or with her. Since I obviously couldn't answer such a question on television, I asked her to leave her name and I would call her. This might be an interesting case, was my thought at the time; and it culminated in several interviews.

When I first talked to her in my office I asked her why she evaluated herself as having a strong personality. She was very bright and verbally fluent, and she said that she felt that a strong person had the following characteristics: high goals (high level of aspiration); high achievement—she had an advance degree in accounting and held a responsible position at management level; high capacity for psychologically and emotionally difficult work; as well as a high level of social dominance ("Nobody, and I mean *nobody* can push me around").

She said that she had had two years of psychotherapy with a psychoanalyst who told her that she was "frigid," and that it might take a long time in therapy (maybe five years or so) to find out why and correct it. She had consulted the psychiatrist because at age twenty-eight she was beginning to worry: she wanted to raise a family.

She was attracted to men and they were to her. But she said, "Nothing good ever happens. I go to bed with them a few times and that's it—a complete waste of time. The men quickly lose interest in me—they feel defeated, I guess, because they can't turn me on."

I asked her if this kind of thing happened frequently. Her answer surprised me: "I couldn't begin to count the number of men I've had affairs with. The longest lasted about one month. I kept going from man to man, hoping to find *someone* that I can make it with."

What really perplexed her was why she was attracted to men so strongly when sex always turned out to be an unrewarding, frustrating experience. It might appear reasonable to believe that her strong interest in men and her lengthy list of sexual encounters meant that she possessed as strong a sexual drive as she possessed a strong personality, even though she said that sex was "nothing" to her. And in fact, in other cases, I had found that one may indeed possess a strong sexual drive while at the same time experiencing failure and frustration in seeking to gratify that drive.

The young woman's problem was not unlike that of one of our earlier research patients, a twenty-three-year-old male, whose problem was that he could rarely complete sexual intercourse. "I get physically tired after thirty minutes or so, and give up. Some women who know this about me won't let me touch them. They say it's exhausting and painful."

The first clue I received about what was possibly involved here came when our blood and odor tests showed him to be a very slow oxidizer—a state which affects many aspects of one's total being. A person in a "slow oxidizing state" is much less sensitive to *pain* than she or he would be if in a "fast oxidizing state." One's pain thresholds go *up* when one's oxidation rate goes *down*. This particular male patient told me that dentists drilled his teeth and also extracted them *without* injecting the pain-deadening Novocaine.

As a rule, a slow oxidizer is less sensitive to all psychological stimuli: noises that bother others they don't even notice; hard knocks (which show up as purple bruises a day later) are virtually ignored; social slights or even direct personal insults are simply brushed off; "sad" music isn't sad; a dented fender on a new car (that one notices after a brief stop at the market) brings neither fleeting thoughts on the futility of life nor the need for a stiff drink.

Further, and directly to the point we are considering, failure to respond to sexual stimulation, the slow oxidizer is a very slow reactor to all the phases of lovemaking.

Having had experience with a number of male patients who had this kind of difficulty, I expected—and found—the bright, dominant young woman executive was a typically insensitive slow oxidizer.

Although most cases of psychochemical imbalance that defy treatment involve slow oxidation, this young woman was able—over a period of eight months—to achieve a relatively "normal" biochemical balance. At the start of the orthonutritional treatment, her Psychochemical Odor score was 32 slow, while after eight months her score was only 8 slow. She was still oriented toward the slow side. This, however, is generally characteristic of highly motivated, achievement-type personalities. But the most notable psychological change that followed the shift in biochemical balance was that she subsequently married, and a year later had a child.

Although I have been using slow oxidizers as examples of impaired sexuality, I have mentioned that any wide deviation from normal biochemical functioning entails sexual difficulties. At the other end of the psychochemical scale, the fast oxidizer is hypersensitive, frequently responding with pain instead of pleasure to sexual stimulation. The following case history of a young married woman (age twenty-six) with two children (aged three and five) is typical.

This research patient was the wife of the director of a medical laboratory which did some of our tests. I was surprised when the director asked me if we could talk about something personal. It seems that he had been questioning some of our research patients about the orthonutritional program, and about the results we were getting. Apparently what he heard satisfied him, and so I asked him to come over for a conversation. Among other things, he told me:

"My wife and I have been married for about six years, and

each year, it seems, our sex life gets less. My wife says she's 'too tired'; 'has a headache'; 'the children have just about driven me crazy all day'; 'I didn't sleep well last night'; 'I'm just about to menstruate'; or 'I'm just getting over my period.'

"Even when she consents, it seems to me that there's nothing in it for her, although she tries to put on a good act. This has got to the point where I feel guilty in even approaching her."

He wanted to know whether I thought her problem could be biochemical. We had a brief discussion of some of the psychological complexities that might be involved—far too many even to enumerate here.

I told him, however, that regardless of the number of psychological possibilities there might be for her behavior, a good place to start would be to *rule out*—if possible—any difficulties that might have biochemical origins.

I took this approach because almost two-thirds of our women research patients who had sexual complaints had previously had "sex therapy," "marriage counseling," or "psychotherapy" of some kind, and in these cases such counseling had been of little or no value, simply because their problems were biochemical, not psychological.

Of course, this is not to dismiss the possible usefulness of psychotherapy in curing sexual disorders. There are two basic types of behavior: *learned* and *psychochemical*. Responses which have been taught, such as "sex is dirty," may, under proper psychotherapy, be unlearned. Psychochemical responses have not been taught. They are the result of experience. "Sex is a big nothing as far as I am concerned" would be a good example. This response can be turned around by psychochemical treatment which increases one's sexual energy, so that the individual now says that sex is rewarding and fulfilling.

No amount of talking about sex can increase one's hormone levels. I do not doubt the value and importance of counseling—

indeed, in many cases, the *necessity*—where the problem is one of psychological adjustment; for many, such counseling is the sole and proper treatment: unlearning attitudes and behavior patterns that are self-destructive.

The problem is to discover which treatment is best for a given individual. From a practical point of view, it seems only reasonable to begin with the treatment which is the easiest, cheapest, and quickest to assess: the psychochemical one.

Here is what Mrs. S., the laboratory director's wife, told me:

"I *always* have a headache of some kind. Sometimes it's just sort of a suggestion in the background—but it's there. My husband dismisses it as 'nerves.'

"Most of the time I'm too tired to even *live*. I wake up tired; by bedtime I'm dead. I ache all over, especially my throbbing head. My husband says he doesn't know what a headache is— he's never had one. Also, he's very strong. He never seems to get tired, and of course he's interested in sex.

"I definitely am *not;* who needs it? I didn't feel this way before I had children. If I ever get pregnant again I just hope someone would shoot me.

"Will you please tell my husband that I'm simply too *tired* for sex?"

Mrs. S. turned out to be a very fast oxidizer. Her Psychochemical Test score was 48 fast. This is the maximum score possible on the test, and goes a long way toward explaining Mrs. S.'s fatigue, headaches, and lack of sexual interest.

Her blood tests were typical for very fast oxidizers, and a nutritional survey we asked her to complete (noting everything she ate for two weeks) revealed a likely source of much of her trouble. As is generally the case with fast oxidizers, she ironically chose the things to eat that made her and kept her *sick*. There is really no other word for it, for Mrs. S. was really suffering, while all the time her physician kept telling her there was nothing at all wrong with her—just "nerves." It was a long, slow climb for Mrs. S. to regain her full strength, but she did. And then some! After being on the orthonutritional program for ten months, she left her husband. A year later she married an affluent automobile dealer from Beverly Hills. I should add that Mrs. S. was a former beauty-contest winner and model, who would cause most men to turn around for another look.

When personality changes begin to appear in patients as a result of improved energy production, their perceptions of others frequently change. To take another example, an almost impotent man told me that once he regained a strong sex drive his wife no longer looked the same or appealed to him as a sex object: "She just looks different. I can't quite put it into words. But her face seems to have a different shape. I don't know whether I have or even both of us have changed." It should be emphasized that this man (age forty-five) had recently married a much younger woman (age twenty-two) and had previously shown little sexual interest in her. He married her when his energies were at a very low point, and having seen the women who appealed to him after treatment, I doubt he would have married the young woman at all had he been functioning at an optimum level. Eventually, he obtained a divorce and soon remarried a totally different type of woman—very Hollywood Boulevard.

The general physical and psychological hypersensitivity of fast oxidizers, which makes sex painful for women, makes it virtually impossible for men. Here is the way one hears about it from the female viewpoint:

"Part of our marriage trouble is sex. My husband is through before I even begin to get warmed up."

Medically this male problem is called "premature ejaculation," but what is literally involved is the heightened sensitivity to *all* incoming psychological stimuli which is characteristic of fast oxidizers. In men this translates into the inability to sustain sexual intercourse because the ultimate psychological intensity of sexual contact is so quickly reached.

I earlier remarked that one's pain thresholds go up when one's oxidation rate goes down. Thus the slower one's oxidation rate, the more pain one can tolerate. This rule applies as well to one's "pleasure thresholds." If I can slow down the rate at which a person is burning oxygen, I can thereby also increase the amount of stimulation necessary to evoke a pleasurable response. The psychological reactions to both painful *and* pleasurable stimuli are delayed when one is in the slow oxidation state. Consequently, one remedy for "premature ejaculation" is to decrease the male patient's general sensitivity to psychological stimuli by decreasing his oxidation rate through personalized orthonutrition.

We earlier listed four psychochemical types: fast, slow, variable oxidizers, and suboxidizers. Up to this point our consideration of personality strength and sexual activity has concentrated on the most common of these types—the fast and slow oxidizers. These are persons who are quite definitely out of biochemical balance, showing differences in Psychochemical Odor Test scores above 16 points (either fast or slow).

In contrast, suboxidizers are not out of biochemical balance. Their scores on the Psychochemical Odor Test are not more than 4 points (either fast or slow), which is what biochemically "normal" people score.

Consequently, the Psychochemical Odor Test does not discriminate between suboxidizers and normal people. Psychological criteria are needed for this purpose. The following are the principal personality characteristics of suboxidizers*:

---

* For a more detailed discussion of this problem, see *Nutrition and Your Mind* (Harper & Row, pages 69–70; Bantam ed., pages 85–86).

Lack of self-confidence
Psychological defensiveness
General apathy
Unsociability
Pessimism
Indecisiveness
Lack of perseverance
Unfavorable self-image
Low motivation

The term "inadequate personality" is often used by psychologists to describe this type of person. Since these same personality traits are also found among fast, slow, and variable oxidizers, they alone cannot be used for classifying a patient. This must be done by *exclusion:* by use of the Psychochemical Odor Test one can exclude the possibility that the patient in question is either a fast, slow, or variable oxidizer, and conclude that he is therefore a suboxidizer.

There is a tendency in the psychological health sciences to include in the concept "patient" the connotation of "young." However, just because most of those seeking psychological help are on the upswing of life (in their late thirties or early forties) does not mean that older persons don't have some of the same problems that younger ones do, and for the *same reasons.*

Even recognizing this I still feel a little uncomfortable in describing a seventy-five-year-old as having an "inadequate personality." Somehow this sounds ridiculous.

"What," you may ask, "does one expect?"

The implication behind this question is that the phrase "old age" *explains* everything. "No sex interest?" "Confidence gone?" "Don't care about much of anything?"

"Well, you're just *old*, that's all." And of course in many cases that may indeed *be* all, for declining age for many brings declining biochemical potentialities. However, the causes of aging itself are hardly understood. Women on the average experience menopause at age fifty, and men are sometimes described as experiencing a similar decline in hormone production at about the same age. The real question, it seems to me, on the basis of my research experience, is how big a factor suboptimal or incorrect nutrition plays in accelerating changes such as these that one associates with the idea of "growing old." Consider the following case histories:

One morning I answered the telephone and at first heard sort of a suppressed giggle—it was my secretary. She said, "There's a man here who says he wants to see the 'sex doctor.' "

I told her to find the name of the doctor the visitor was looking for, since he had obviously entered the wrong door. At that time my office was in a rather large medical complex containing dozens of medical suites.

She soon called back, saying the man insisted he was in the right office. "He won't leave. Couldn't you just talk to him briefly to straighten the matter out?"

I'm glad I was free at the moment and said "yes." I learned a lot.

The unknown visitor wore overalls, was quite tan from outdoor work, and had light blue eyes that contrasted nicely with his white hair.

He diffidently asked me if I was the doctor who "fixed sex." He seemed embarrassed, looking past me when he spoke the words "fixed sex."

Although by then I had a backlog of several dozen cases in which impotence and frigidity had vanished as a result of the orthonutritional treatment, all of these cases were of persons of much younger age (the oldest was fifty-three). Furthermore, the revival of sexual interest and activity in these cases had not been my goal. I would never have dreamed of trying to run a research program designed to understand and treat problems of a sexual nature.

But I was more than a little curious both about this caller—he was obviously an "old" man—and about where he had got my name in connection with sexual disturbances. So I began to question him about his background and about how he came to believe I was someone who could help him. But my direct questions received no answers. He had a story to tell:

He had been married forty years to a "hard woman." He was seventy-five and she was seventy. This woman ran a tight ship. After dinner he was not allowed to sit in the living room: he was too dirty. Instead, he had a shop in the garage. There was a good chair and a television set in the shop. He had spent almost every evening alone in the garage for "upwards of twenty years"—except Thanksgiving and Christmas evenings, when he was allowed in the house.

"But," he said, "lately I've been feeling a little lonely, and I started taking a walk each evening. I go down the long block on which we live, cross the street, and walk back. My wife comes out on the front porch and watches me until I'm out of sight. She's never said anything."

Well, on one of these walks he got into a conversation with a "nice lady" who was generally out watering her plants when he passed her house. Since he was a gardener, they had a common interest, but soon they weren't talking about plants and flowers.

She invited him in and gave him coffee and cake "made with her own hands." She was sixty.

He finally got to the point. They liked each other, and she was so upset when she heard that he had been "treated like a dog" for all those years that she asked him to come live with her. "And," he added, "if I do, I'll need some help about sex."

This sad story really got to me. I would have done anything to be able to help him. I simply couldn't bring myself to tell him what I thought was the truth—namely, that his request for sexual rehabilitation was a hopeless proposition.

Instead, I decided to approach his problem with our routine tests, which he was eager to take. Since I had never had a research patient anywhere near his age, I had no idea what to expect.

Fortunately, all of the tests put him in the suboxidizer category, so he could eat a normal diet, only increasing the amount of protein. I gave him a month's supply of the vitamin-mineral supplement for suboxidizers, telling him to start with the maximum intake amd come back in a month.

It was six weeks, however, before he returned. He told me that he hadn't come back before since the treatment seemed to have solved his problem. "But," he said, "I found that ten or twelve days after I'd taken all those pills, and I didn't have any more, well—the sex problem returned. I guess I just need those pills."

Was this seventy-five-year-old's impotence—he said he had stopped thinking about sex twenty-five years ago—due to irreversible glandular changes that simply occurred with the passage of time? Or were his tissues being deprived of the nutritional substances they needed to make hormones?

Consider another example:

A fifty-five-year-old married woman was referred to me by a physician friend who told me that she had "all sorts of vague complaints" that did not fit into any medical category he knew of. He thought a nutritional boost might possibly help, and there was no point in sending her to another physician.

She was a suboxidizer, and she certainly exhibited the psychological characteristics of one—she had an "inadequate personality." She had two married daughters, and had been through menopause ten years earlier (at age forty-five).

Since she was not a participant in a formal research group° she was not given a placebo trial period, but was directly placed on the orthonutritional program for suboxidizers. At the end of one month she returned, reporting some general improvement in energy and activity level. This gradual improvement continued for another two months.

Then I received a telephone call from the physician who had referred her to me. He sounded angry. "What the devil are you giving to Mrs. R.? Two weeks ago she came to see me and she was in a panic: vaginal bleeding, fear of cancer. We have checked her thoroughly and have found nothing wrong. She simply appears to be *menstruating.*"

He suspected that we were giving her hormones as part of her treatment. When I told him most emphatically we were not, he said he couldn't believe that intensive nutritional therapy could "reverse the normal aging process in women."

Well, that is the question we are asking: what indeed is the "normal aging process"?

I personally was not altogether surprised that this fifty-five-year-old post-menopausal patient began menstruating. This phenomenon had been reported to me countless times. However, these former patients had all been "young"—from sixteen to forty-five, and none had been through what is called "menopause."

° Nor was the seventy-five-year-old male patient just described.

I have found that failure to menstruate and irregular periods are *characteristic* of patients who are not functioning at a normal or optimal biochemical level from a nutritional standpoint. Virtually all such patients are not only generally undernourished—that is, on the wrong diet for their particular modes of metabolism—but as a consequence they are overstressed. They simply cannot handle a "normal" day's burden without caving in. They are not only unable to produce the energy they need, but they are also unable to make new cells rapidly enough to keep their bodies functioning at an optimal level.

One of the first places failure to produce new cells normally shows up in women is the menstrual cycle: missed periods. In men it is loss of libido: sexual interest and potency require an ample ability to produce hormones, which are protein structures that are literally manufactured from the food one eats.

In concluding this brief discussion of the relationships between orthonutrition, personality, and sex I wish to emphasize comments I have made on their interrelation at the beginning of this chapter.

Since all hormones are synthesized by glands in the body from biochemicals that one obtains from one's dietary intake, any alteration in nutrition affects one's hormone production. Consequently, when we place a *mis*nourished person on a food and supplement intake that meets his or her optimum and unique needs, hormone production increases, with consequent changes in personality strength, including increased interest in sex and sexual activity.

Even though my research goals are not directly related to sex, the problem arises because sex is such an integral characteristic of a patient's personality strength.

I have never contemplated a controlled study of the effects of orthonutrition on sexual attitudes and behavior. This by all means ought to be done by scientists whose principal field of interest is human sexuality.

My justification for including uncontrolled case history material is to call attention to this urgent and totally neglected research area, in the hope that others may think twice before they pronounce a patient "frigid" or "impotent," and say that these problems are "psychological" and largely untreatable.

7

The Psychochemical Odor Test
as a Guide to Orthonutrition

This test, used together with the suggested diets and nutritional supplements to be described in this chapter, will allow one to increase his or her personality strength, providing the following conditions are also being met: one has adequate rest, minimum stress, regular exercise. One should work to discover and eliminate situations and behavior that cause stress. In addition, one should schedule a program of regular periods of strenuous exercise, such as *brisk* walking, jogging, swimming—in short, physical activity that increases one's oxygen consumption and therefore capacity.

With the exception of the slow oxidizers, virtually all those I have interviewed and tested who said that they considered themselves to be "normal, healthy, and well nourished" still recorded abnormal scores on this test. They were either burning starches and sugars too fast, thus depriving themselves of the major sources of energy production in the tissues (protein and fat), or burning blood sugar too slowly, which also deprives one of the full food energy available in these items. Neither protein nor fat can be utilized fully unless adequate amounts of carbohydrate are being provided. (Those readers who have not read *Nutrition and Your Mind* might turn to the general discussion there in Chapter V on how the body makes energy from food.)

Virtually all of the subjects who participated in the research upon which this book is based were psychologically "normal": they had normal profiles on the Minnesota Multiphasic Personality Inventory, and most of them had never sought psychological or psychiatric help. Few of them registered very high or very low on the Psychochemical Odor Test. Such "normal" subjects are very hard to identify on blood tests, while those with psychological problems are easily identified on the group of blood tests described in the Appendix of *Nutrition and Your Mind*. On the other hand, the Psychochemical Odor Test reliably distinguishes between fast and slow oxidizers who are psychologically "normal" but are not functioning at their full capacities. The test also isolates individuals with severe psychological difficulties. But the following dietary and nutritional supplementary suggestions are particularly directed to the ostensibly "normal" group.

To repeat, one's goal in using the test, the diets, and the supplements is to *attain* and *maintain* optimum biochemical balance, together with the nutritional intake that will produce the energy output which provides the vigor for one's personality strength.

Suboxidizers (0-4, fast or slow) eat a "normal" diet," providing they obtain an optimum protein intake, plus an intake of whole-grain bread or cereals, together with sufficient vegetables and fruit to make up their caloric needs which are not provided for by their protein intake. They should be careful neither to gain nor to lose weight, and to check frequently to see that their Psychochemical Odor Test score remains at 0-4, fast or slow. In addition, they should take the following mineral-and-vitamin supplement of which each capsule contains:

Vitamin A (palmitate)	10,000 I.U.
Vitamin E (mixed tocopherols)	200 I.U.
Vitamin B_{12}	50 mcg.
Niacinamide	200 mg.
Pantothenate	50 mg.
Vitamin C	200 mg.
Vitamin B_1	10 mg.
Vitamin B_2	10 mg.
Vitamin B_6	10 mg.
PABA (para-amino benzoic acid)	25 mg.
Choline	200 mg.
Inositol	160 mg.
Calcium	220 mg.
Phosphate	150 mg.
Iodine	0.15 mg.
Zinc (sulfate)	5 mg.
Magnesium	100 mg.
Ferrous (sulfate)	20 mg.

The recommended intake for suboxidizers is two capsules after breakfast and two capsules after lunch (total daily intake: four capsules). For some individuals, an added capsule after dinner increases their energy the following day. It is best to vary your intake to see what works best for you. On the other hand, about 98 percent of our suboxidizer research patients responded best at an intake of four capsules daily, taken as directed above.

Owing to the simplified manner in which the test is constructed, each psychochemical type is limited by a small spread of scores: the highest score for suboxidizers is 4, while this same number is the lowest score for both fast and slow oxidizers. The individual must *adjust* his or her nutritional intake on the basis of the direction (either fast or slow) his or her scores tend to run.

For example, if a suboxidizer scores 4 fast with an occasional 8 or even 12 he or she would be considered a mild fast oxidizer (scores 4-16 fast). Such individuals should test the diet and supplement recommended for mild fast oxidizers: it might be more effective than the program recommended for suboxidizers.

Variable oxidizers should select their food and food supplements on the basis of an odor test score taken before breakfast. They may have to test themselves again later in the day, depending upon their homeostatic stability. Fortunately there appear to be very few variable oxidizers around like Professor Carter (Chapter 2). He had to carry an odor kit with him for over a year before he achieved a normal biochemical balance.

Those who have an unpredictable reaction to what they eat should always check their test scores before eating meals and taking food supplements. By doing this faithfully, they can achieve a normal biochemical balance and an optimum output of mental, emotional, and physical energy.

ORTHONUTRITION FOR NORMAL AND SUBOXIDIZERS (0-4, FAST OR SLOW)

You calculate optimum protein intake by dividing your "ideal weight" by the number 15, as I have mentioned earlier. The resulting figure is the number of ounces of *lean* meat (all kinds), chicken, turkey, and fish to be eaten each day°. This figure will meet or slightly exceed the recommended allowances suggested by the National Research Council.

° One medium-sized egg or one cup of milk may be substituted for one ounce of meat.

What is your ideal weight? If you are healthy, suffering from no medical condition (such as diabetes) that requires medical supervision, your ideal weight is what *you* want to weigh. As a matter of fact, no scientist can say what an ideal or a correct weight is for any given individual. What diet books and charts give in their tables is figures drawn from *averages* of millions of people; these averages are derived principally from life-insurance statistics, based upon such variables as sex, height, age, and weight as related to longevity. Since the number of calories obtained in this manner is an *average,* it need not be suitable to your own optimum health. As a matter of scientific fact, the whole subject of who should weigh what is largely a medical enigma. Many persons cannot lose weight on a 500-calories-per-day diet, when by biochemical standards such a diet should result in a weight loss of one pound per week (one pound of body weight equaling 3,500 calories).

The calories from the protein you consume determine how much other food you require. Carbohydrates, such as whole-grain cereals and bread, vegetables and fruit (not canned with added sugar), are *equally as important* to one's health as are the protein and fat (also essential) one consumes. The importance of fat in the diet, both saturated (meat fat) and unsaturated (vegetable and fish oils), is that the body cannot assimilate and use certain very important vitamins (A, D, K, and E) in the absence of the fatty acids in meat and milk, for example, to transport these vitamins through the intestinal wall and carry them in the blood to where they are needed in the tissues.

In addition to knowing how many ounces of protein foods you need per day, you should also balance or vary these foods:

One-third of your protein should be *"neutral proteins"*: eggs, cheese, milk, cereal, and/or vegetable proteins in combinations that nutritionally approximate the complete proteins found in meat, fowl, etc.°

Two-thirds of your protein should come from complete proteins such as meat (any kind), fish, and fowl.

The carbohydrates (sugars and starches) you consume should come from three sources. Part of it should be derived from whole-grain (that is, *unrefined*) breads and cereals. These provide fiber (bulk) in the diet, which is *essential* to good nutrition, as well as calories, vitamins, and minerals. In addition to cereals, vegetables provide needed carbohydrates, vitamins, and minerals. The third source of carbohydrates is fruit, preferably whole fruit, not juice (unless one also drinks the pulp in the juice). Refined sugars, such as those obtained from sugar cane or sugar beets, ideally should be avoided completely. They are absorbed and oxidized too fast, and they also increase the body's needs for the vitamins and minerals necessary to utilize them. The trouble with refined sugars is that they enter the blood almost immediately; they are too concentrated and metabolize too fast. This same objection may be applied to *any* concentrated source of sugar: honey, raw sugar, dates, raisins, etc. Persons substituting honey or raw sugar for the white sugar in the sugar bowl are simply deceiving themselves if they think that what they are feeding themselves is an improvement over white sugar. The key to this whole problem is the *concentration* of sugar: it provides too many calories too quickly, thus *displacing more nutritious*

° The subject of how to combine vegetables and cereals proportionately to roughly equate animal protein is far too complex to discuss here. It involves the eight essential amino acids that the body cannot synthesize, and which amino acids have to be provided in the *right proportions*. For those who have the time and patience, *this can be rewarding*. What you require, however, is a book on vegetarianism. Your library or bookstore will have them. You may also write to Loma Linda University, Riverside, California 92505. They distribute literature on this subject without charge.

foods from the diet. Consequently, concentrated sweets, including candy and pastry, should be used *sparingly,* certainly not more than fifty calories per day. If you want something sweet to eat, it should be a piece of low-calorie fruit, such as a slice of melon, a small apple, or an orange.

If one's goal is orthonutrition, meaning optimum mental and physical strength, then sugars should play a very small role in one's total daily caloric intake. If used to excess they *diminish* one's energy output, which is the very last thing we are aiming at.

Sub- and normal oxidizers have freedom of choice of proteins, cereals, vegetables, and fruit. They only must make sure to (1) get the protein amount appropriate to their weight; (2) eat whole-grain breads and cereals; (3) eat fresh vegetables and fruit as often as possible; and (4) avoid concentrated sweets of any kind. Finally, and *most important*, one should take the recommended nutritional supplement *regularly:* NEVER MISS A DAY!

ORTHONUTRITION FOR FAST OXIDIZERS

For orthonutritional purposes, fast oxidizers can be divided into two categories. Those who score 4-16. And those who score 16-32. The allowed lunch foods and lunch menus are the same for both categories. Breakfasts and dinners, however, differ.

ALLOWED BREAKFAST FOODS FOR FAST OXIDIZERS (4–16)

1. Proteins
  Ground lean meat patty (beef or veal)
  Ham slice
  Ham and egg omelet

Lox or herring
Minute steak
Corned beef hash
  (with egg, if desired)

2. *Carbohydrates*
    Oatmeal with half-and-half
    Whole-grain toast with butter
    Whole-wheat English muffin with butter

3. *Beverages*
    Decaffeinated coffee
    Hot tea with cream (with sugar substitute if available; if not, 1 level teaspoon sugar [20 calories])
    Small (6-ounce) glass tomato juice

4. *No fruit*

TYPICAL BREAKFAST, FAST OXIDIZER (4–16)

Beverage: Small glass of tomato juice or *decaffeinated coffee with cream*
Protein: Ham omelet made with one egg only; the greater portion of one's protein here should come from chopped lean ham; the egg may be beaten with a small amount of cream (sufficient to provide the bulk to incorporate the ham in the omelet)
Carbohydrates: Whole-grain toast with butter

ALLOWED BREAKFAST FOODS FOR FAST OXIDIZERS (16–32)

1. *Proteins*
    Meat patty (lamb or pork)
    Link sausages
    Liver with bacon

Smoked salmon or herring
Pork chop(s)
Lamb chop(s)

2. Carbohydrates
Hash-browned potato patty
Whole-grain toast with butter
Whole-grain English muffin with butter

3. Beverages
Hot chocolate made with unsweetened chocolate (not cocoa) and half-and-half with whole milk (equal portions), sweetened to taste
Decaffeinated coffee with cream

TYPICAL BREAKFAST, FAST OXIDIZER (16–32)

Beverage: Decaffeinated coffee with cream
Protein: Link sausages
Carbohydrates: Hash-browned potato patty
Whole-grain toast with butter

ALLOWED LUNCH FOODS FOR FAST OXIDIZERS (4–16 OR 16–32)

1. Proteins
Sliced roast meat (beef or ham), with gravy
Cheeseburger with mayonnaise; no catsup or onion; Russian dressing allowed, if made with mayonnaise and catsup only
Salmon (canned or fresh)
Deep-fried seafood (shrimp, scallops, oysters)
Grilled ham-and-cheese sandwich on whole-wheat bread
Roast-beef hash with gravy
Ham-and-lima-bean casserole

2. Soups
Cream of spinach, split pea, navy bean, corn or clam chowder

3. Carbohydrates
Beans
Peas
Corn
Creamed potatoes with cheese
(No onions, peppers, cucumbers, pickles, lettuce; one or two slices
    of ripe tomato permitted)
Cornbread with butter
Whole-grain bread or roll with butter

4. Beverages
Tea, cold or hot, with cream
Decaffeinated coffee, cold or hot, with cream

5. Desserts
Jello with whipped cream
Cheesecake (SMALL slice)

TYPICAL LUNCH, FAST OXIDIZER (4–16 OR 16–32)

Beverage: Decaffeinated coffee or tea with cream
Soup: Split pea
Protein: Roast meat with gravy
Carbohydrates: Creamed potatoes with cheese
Whole-grain roll or bread with butter
Dessert: Jello with whipped cream

ALLOWED DINNER FOODS FOR FAST OXIDIZERS (4–16)

1. Proteins
Roast or fried chicken, leg and thigh only
Tuna casserole made with half-and-half and egg noodles

Beef or veal stew (no onions)
Pork-and-bean casserole (no sugar, small amount of catsup; garlic
    powder seasoning allowed)
Pot roast of beef cooked with potatoes
Veal or pork chops

2. Carbohydrates
Snap beans with bacon bits
Cauliflower (no cabbage or sprouts)
Creamed carrots
Baked potato with butter
Peas
Corn (fresh with butter, or frozen, unsweetened with butter)

3. Beverages
Decaffeinated coffee or tea with cream

4. Desserts
Sliced banana with cream
Small serving of chocolate pudding made with unsweetened
    chocolate and cream

TYPICAL DINNER, FAST OXIDIZER (4–16)

Beverage: Decaffeinated coffee or tea with cream
Protein: Pot roast of beef cooked with potatoes and served with gravy
    (lamb or veal stew optional)
Carbohydrates: Snap beans with bacon bits
Cornbread or muffins with butter
Dessert: Sliced small banana with whipped cream

ALLOWED DINNER FOODS FOR FAST OXIDIZERS (16–32)

1. Proteins
Roast turkey, leg and thigh only

Short ribs of beef with pan-cooked potatoes
Roast veal or lamb
Veal chops
Lamb chops
Corned beef served with creamed cauliflower
Liver with bacon
Seafood plate: scallops, shrimp, abalone, lobster; tartar sauce made with no onion, no sweet pickles but with dill pickle bits and garlic seasoning (not fresh garlic)
Meat loaf made from combined pork, veal, beef, served with mashed potatoes; garlic seasoning. Serve with creamed pan gravy

2. Carbohydrates
Creamed chopped spinach
Asparagus
Cauliflower
Lentils
Baked potato with butter
Lima beans cooked with ham hocks

3. Beverages
Decaffeinated coffee or tea with cream

4. Desserts
Cheesecake
Small, rich custard pudding with whipped cream

TYPICAL DINNER, FAST OXIDIZER (16–32)

Beverage: Decaffeinated coffee or tea with cream
Protein: Short ribs of beef with pan-fried potatoes
Carbohydrates: Creamed cauliflower
Whole-grain muffins or bread with butter
Dessert: Small chocolate pudding with whipped cream

ORTHONUTRITION FOR SLOW OXIDIZERS

Slow oxidizers may also be broken up into the categories 4-16 and 16-32. However, *their* allowed lunch foods are not the same.

ALLOWED BREAKFAST FOODS FOR SLOW OXIDIZERS (4–16)

1. *Proteins*
   Eggs, any style (the number of eggs depending upon one's protein requirements)
   Cereals: rice, wheat, or corn, cold or hot, served with low-fat milk and fruit, if desired°

2. *Carbohydrates*
   Any fresh fruit available (seasonally)

3. *Beverages*
   Low-fat milk
   Buttermilk
   Tomato, orange, or grapefruit juice (no grape, cranberry, or apple juice)
   Black coffee (no cream or sugar)
   Tea (slightly sweetened with sugar if desired)

TYPICAL BREAKFAST, SLOW OXIDIZER (4–16)

Beverage: Fresh orange juice (if available); otherwise reconstituted frozen juice
Coffee

° There is one dry cereal on the market, prepared from a mixture of grains to constitute a complete protein, comparable to animal protein. The label states that it contains 40 percent complete protein (the best sources of animal protein rarely contain 25 percent). Although the cereal manufacturers rate low for nutrition generally, I feel it is only fair to mention one that is good: Kellogg's Concentrate.

Protein: Two soft-boiled eggs (three if your protein requirements indicate three)
Carbohydrates: Toasted whole-wheat English muffin with corn-oil or safflower-oil margarine (no *butter)*

ALLOWED BREAKFAST FOODS FOR SLOW OXIDIZERS (16–32)

1. *Proteins*
Cereals: Hot—Cream of Wheat or Cream of Rice
Cold—Rice Krispies°
  (Either served with skim milk)
Yogurt

2. *Carbohydrates*
White toast with margarine
Graham crackers (with low-fat milk)
Fresh fruit: grapefruit, oranges, melon, berries (any kind), apple(s)

3. *Beverages*
Grapefruit juice (unsweetened)
Buttermilk
Tea with lemon (slightly sweetened if desired)
Skim milk (flavored with vanilla and teaspoon of sugar if desired)

TYPICAL BREAKFAST, SLOW OXIDIZER (16–32)

Beverage: Grapefruit juice
Protein: Hot Cream of Wheat with low-fat milk
Carbohydrates: Fresh fruit
Tea with lemon, sweetened if desired

° With the exception of Kellogg's Concentrate, the protein from hot or cold cereals is contained in the milk with which they are served. In general, the 16–32 slow oxidizer must obtain his breakfast protein from milk and/or yogurt. However, Kellogg's Concentrate is too heavy in protein for very slow oxidizers (16–32). It may, however, be combined half and half with another dry cereal to increase protein, when needed.

ALLOWED LUNCH FOODS FOR SLOW OXIDIZERS (4–16)

1. *Proteins*
   Cottage cheese with lettuce and fruit
   Fillet of sole (or any other "light" fish)
   Stuffed bell pepper with chicken or egg salad
   Chicken salad (white meat)
   Chef's salad (mixed greens with small strips of cheese and ham)
   Egg-salad sandwich
   "Fishburger"
   Minced-ham omelet

2. *Salads*
   Tomato aspic
   Lettuce with oil-and-vinegar dressing
   Cole slaw
   Potato salad

3. *Soups*
   Chicken broth with rice
   Mixed vegetable soup
   French onion soup

4. *Vegetables*
   All except *asparagus, spinach, cauliflower, lentils, beans, peas*

5. *Other carbohydrates*
   All fruit except avocados

6. *Beverages*
   Tea, black coffee, buttermilk, low-fat milk, any fruit or vegetable
   drink

7. *Desserts*
   Fresh fruit, fruit jello, orange/lemon/or raspberry sherbet

TYPICAL LUNCH, SLOW OXIDIZER (4–16)

Beverage: Black coffee
Soup: Vegetable
Protein: Minced-ham omelet
Vegetable: Broccoli
Dessert: Orange sherbet

ALLOWED LUNCH FOODS FOR SLOW OXIDIZERS (16–32)

1. *Proteins*
Fish (preferably baked or poached): sole, cod, halibut, perch, turbot
Mixed vegetable salad with farmer-style cottage cheese, oil-and-vinegar dressing
Breast-of-chicken sandwich, with lettuce, mayonnaise, and mustard
Spanish omelet (with onions, green peppers, and hot sauce)

2. *Soups*
Tomato
Potato (made with low-fat milk)
Potato and leek
Vegetable broth

3. *Salads*
Diced carrots with lettuce
Sliced pickled beets
Waldorf salad
Radish, celery, carrot-stick, pickle-chip plate

4. *Vegetables*
All except asparagus, spinach, cauliflower, lentils, beans, peas, and corn

5. *Other carbohydrates*
All fruit (except avocados)

6. Beverages
Tea with lemon, buttermilk, low-fat milk, any fruit juice (unsweetened)

7. Desserts
Fruit jello, fresh fruit, sherbet

TYPICAL LUNCH, SLOW OXIDIZER (16–32)

Beverage: Tea with lemon, and/or sugar, if desired
Soup: Tomato
Protein: Spanish omelet (the number of eggs used determined by your protein requirement)
Vegetables: Radish, celery, carrot-stick, and pickle-chip plate. Boiled banana squash (mashed or sliced) with margarine
Dessert: Lemon aspic

ALLOWED DINNER FOODS FOR SLOW OXIDIZERS (16–32)

1. Proteins
Baked breast of chicken with dressing (include onions, celery, parsley, poultry seasoning with toasted cubes of white bread; margarine for fat)
Baked breast of turkey with dressing (same dressing described above, adding fresh green peppers if desired)
Baked halibut with lemon (or any fresh fish)
Cottage cheese, yogurt, and fruit, combined in a salad, yogurt providing the dressing
Cold plate: sliced lean boiled ham, jack cheese, deviled egg, carrot and celery sticks, on bed of lettuce with oil-and-vinegar dressing (potato salad optional)

2. Soups
Chicken broth with rice and okra
Turkey broth with rice and okra

Mixed vegetable
French onion

3. *Salads*
Fruit aspic
Vegetable aspic
Mixed lettuce with tomato slices and cucumber slices
Mixed fresh fruit salad

4. *Vegetables*
All except asparagus, spinach, cauliflower, lentils, beans, peas, and corn

5. *Other carbohydrates*
All fruit (except avocados)

6. *Beverages*
Tea with lemon, slightly sweetened if desired
Lemonade
Low-fat milk with added chocolate flavoring

7. *Desserts*
Fresh fruit, as desired

TYPICAL DINNER, SLOW OXIDIZER (16–32)

Soup: French onion soup
Proteins: Baked breast of chicken with dressing
Vegetables: Broccoli
Vegetable aspic
Dessert: Raspberry sherbet
Beverage: Tea with lemon, slightly sweetened

SUMMARY OF NUTRITIONAL SUPPLEMENTS FOR
SUBOXIDIZERS, FAST OXIDIZERS (4–16 AND 16–32),
AND SLOW OXIDIZERS (4–16 AND 16–32)

1. *Suboxidizer Daily Supplement: One after each meal (three per day)*

Vitamin A (palmitate)	10,000 I.U.
Vitamin E (mixed tocopherols)	200 I.U.
Vitamin B_1	10 mg.
Vitamin B_2	10 mg.
Vitamin B_6	10 mg.
Vitamin B_{12}	50 mcg.
Niacinamide	200 mg.
Pantothenate	50 mg.
PABA	25 mg.
Vitamin C	200 mg.
Choline	200 mg.
Inositol	160 mg.
Calcium	220 mg.
Phosphate	150 mg.
Iodine	0.05 mg.
Zinc	5 mg.
Magnesium	100 mg.
Iron (ferrous gluconate)	75 mg.

1. *Fast Oxidizer Basic Formula. Each capsule contains:*

Vitamin A (palmitate)	10,000 I.U.
Vitamin E (mixed tocopherols)	200 I.U.
Vitamin B_{12}	100 mcg.
Vitamin C	200 mg.
Niacinamide	200 mg.
Pantothenate	100 mg.
Choline	200 mg.
Inositol	160 mg.

Calcium	*220 mg.*
Phosphate	*150 mg.*
Iodine	*0.05 mg.*
Zinc sulfate	*7 mg.*

Recommended intakes:

Fast Oxidizers (4–16): Two after breakfast, and two after lunch (total four per day)

Fast Oxidizers (16–32): Two after breakfast, two after lunch, and one after dinner (total five per day)

2. *Slow Oxidizer Basic Formula. Each capsule contains:*

Vitamin A (fish liver oil)	*10,000 I.U.*
Vitamin B_1	*10 mg.*
Vitamin B_2	*10 mg.*
Vitamin B_6	*10 mg.*
Vitamin C	*250 mg.*
Vitamin D	*400 I.U.*
Niacin	*25 mg.*
PABA	*100 mg.*
Potassium citrate	*300 mg.*
Magnesium chloride	*100 mg.*
Copper gluconate	*0.2 mg.*
Ferrous gluconate	*25 mg.*

Recommended intakes:

Slow Oxidizers (4–16): Two after breakfast, and two after lunch (total four per day)

Slow Oxidizers (16–32): Two after breakfast, two after lunch, and one after dinner (total five per day)

A careful reader of the preceding chapters will have noticed a repeating pattern of repetition: I tell you the same thing again and again, perhaps worded slightly differently. *This repetition is not accidental:* my experience with readers of *Nutrition and Your Mind* was both enlightening and discouraging. In the first place I received (and am still receiving) an unbelievable quantity of mail—far beyond anyone's capacity to read, much less answer. I have, however, read several hundred letters, and virtually all of them asked questions or wanted information that was already clearly covered in the book. Consequently, by repetition I have tried to get my message across to even the most casual reader.

Questions will come up, however, concerning specific foods that I have not mentioned. They are not included in the foods listed because I don't know any more about them than does the reader. In this type of situation, I can only suggest that you try the food(s) in question and determine your own reaction.

One final repetition: the goal of using the Psychochemical Odor Test, following the diets, and taking the food supplements is to *attain and keep a normal biochemical balance while providing an optimum intake of the foods you need when you need them.* This is the only way that you can achieve your maximum personality strength and physical endurance. This is *Orthonutrition,* and how to get there is set out in detail in the book you've just read.

Appendix

**A BRIEF SUMMARY OF THE KINDS OF RESEARCH DATA
UPON WHICH THE FOREGOING CHAPTERS ARE BASED**

Three kinds of information were used in assessing the effects of the orthonutritional program on research patients before, during, and at the conclusion of treatment periods: blood tests, psychological tests and rating scales, and the Psychochemical Odor Test.

The following discussion is not intended for the general reader, but for the technically trained therapist or scientist who would like to see the comparison of scores on these variables with changes in behavior and attitudes by the subject's own self-ratings.

The total number of research subjects involved in this experiment was 358. All of these volunteered for the study because of vague symptoms of malaise for which their doctors could find no medical reason: they were all medically "healthy." Still, in the face of this opinion they all expressed the general feeling that "something must be wrong, and I'm not imagining it—regardless of what my doctor says."

The length of time a subject might be under observation varied from three months to two years. By "under observation" I mean that the patients had monthly one-half-hour interviews to review what they were doing and how they were progressing. One of the principal reasons that some of the treatment periods were so short was that some patients quickly learned what they were to do and faithfully carried out the recommendations given to them. Also, some individuals (principally the younger, 18-28 years old) responded very quickly to the orthonutritional regimen.

Since this book is intended principally for the general reader rather than for professionals, I will simply present a statistical summary of some of the research results by giving a random sample of the data on one hundred patients, fifty drawn from the fast oxidizer files and fifty drawn from the slow oxidizer files.

Each subject acted as his or her own control, being kept on placebos until he or she reported "no progress," and the self-ratings, blood tests, and Psychochemical Odor Test scores remained unchanged. (The sexually troubled patients described in Chapter 6 were not part of a formal research group. In their cases, controls were not used. I have never contemplated a controlled study of the effects of orthonutrition on sexual attitudes and behavior. This by all means ought to be done by scientists whose principal field of interest is human sexuality. As I have stated above, my justification for including uncontrolled case-history material in this book is to call attention to an urgent and totally neglected research area, in the hope that others may think twice before they pronounce a patient "frigid" or "impotent," and say that these problems are psychological and largely untreatable.)

The total N, 358 (age range 16–52), is the number of research subjects who began the study and completed it. An additional 69 patients started the program and then dropped out—principally while taking placebos. Obviously, these dropouts were not among the patients whose scores appeared in our random sampling. The absence of final assessments on the 69 dropouts does not materially alter the final statistical evaluations, for when

STATISTICAL SUMMARY OF A RANDOM SAMPLE OF ONE HUNDRED RESEARCH PATIENTS, FIFTY FAST OXIDIZERS AND FIFTY SLOW OXIDIZERS ON FIVE PARAMETERS OF EVALUATION

FAST OXIDIZERS N=50

	FASTING BLOOD SUGAR		PLASMA PH		DISSOLVED $CO_2 + H_2CO_3$		PERSONALITY RATINGS*		PSYCHOCHEMICAL ODOR TEST	
	Before	After	Before	After	Before	After	Before	After	Before	After
RANGE	69–82	95–105	7.33–7.48	7.42–7.46	1.00–1.20	1.29–1.35	1.00–9.00	7.00–9.00	12–28	4–12
MEAN	76.20	96.00	7.38	7.44	1.14	1.32	3.8	7.2	20	4
STANDARD ERROR OF THE DIFFERENCE BETWEEN MEANS	3.52		0.02		0.07		1.76		3.29	
SIGNIFICANCE LEVEL	p<.001		p<.001		p<.001		p<.001		p<.001	

SLOW OXIDIZERS N=50

	FASTING BLOOD SUGAR		PLASMA PH		DISSOLVED $CO_2 + H_2CO_3$		PERSONALITY RATINGS*		PSYCHOCHEMICAL ODOR TEST	
	Before	*After*	*Before*	*After*	*Before*	*After*	*Before*	*After*	*Before*	*After*
RANGE	79–87	95–105	7.46–7.50	7.40–7.45	1.18–1.27	1.28–1.35	1.00–4.00	6.00–8.00	12–24	0–12
MEAN	82.00	100.00	7.48	7.42	1.22	1.36	2.80	7.90	17.20	4.80
STANDARD ERROR OF THE DIFFERENCE BETWEEN MEANS	2.60		0.01		0.04		1.13		3.39	
SIGNIFICANCE LEVEL	$p<.001$		$p<.001$		$p<.001$		$p<.001$		$p<.001$	

*For a listing of the items on the subject's own personality ratings see page 138.

137

their beginning and ending scores are entered as being identical (i.e., zero improvement), the final probabilities (significance levels) are not appreciably changed.

Several widely used psychometric instruments were used at the beginning of this experiment. I will not name them, since the following ten-item scale yielded comparable results ($p < .01$) and could be answered by the subject in a very short time and scored in even less time.° Research subjects *do not like* (and frequently will not complete) comprehensive, time-consuming paper-and-pencil tests.

Here are the test items; the subjects rated themselves on an eleven-point scale (0-10). For example a person who was very tolerant of others might score his or herself as 9, while an intolerant person might score 3.

1. *Patience*
2. *Self-confidence*
3. *Aggressiveness*
4. *Self-respect*
5. *Optimism*
6. *Energy level*
7. *Perseverance*
8. *Tolerance of others*
9. *Friendliness*
10. *Happiness*

For the nonscientific reader who would like to have some idea of the meaning of the statistical data on pages 136–137, the significance (or confidence) level of the Psychochemical Odor Test

---

° One other point should be mentioned: since one of the principal aims of this study was to determine the extent, if any, an individual's self-image could be altered through orthonutrition, a patient's own self-rating was considered to be a better index of this than a personality test designed to evaluate a patient for the interviewer. Questions of reliability and validity are also avoided; they are irrelevant.

(p<. 001) is equal to that of the blood tests and personality ratings. Thus it is a valid and reliable indicator of one's nutritional
balance, as represented by one's fasting blood sugar, plasma pH,
total carbon dioxide, and carbonic acid levels.†

---

† For a discussion of this general problem, see *Nutrition and Your Mind* (Harper & Row,
pages 87–94; Bantam paperback edition, pages 106–114).

Editor's Note About the
Origins of This Book

For readers unfamiliar with his earlier book, *Nutrition and Your Mind* (Harper & Row, 1972), diving into these pages may come as something of a shock. Actually, the development of the Psychochemical Odor Test has been almost a lifetime occupation for George Watson, going back to the late 1940s when he held a post-doctoral research fellowship in psychology at the University of Southern California. He was working in the area of odor theory. Because their odor intensities could be controlled, he primarily used water-soluble vitamins, in particular 10-milligram tablets of thiamine hydrochloride. One day, on a whim, he swallowed (with water) one 100-milligram tablet of thiamine. It was late in the afternoon and he was getting fatigued mentally, ready to quit work for the day. But he wanted to see the effect on the odor test scale of the 100 milligrams of thiamine, so he waited about thirty minutes and retested the odor. Not only was it quantitatively beyond the scale, but the odor had changed qualitatively so that it was no longer typical of thiamine at ten milligrams. Watson noticed that he no longer felt quite so tired.

This experience changed his orientation toward the research, and he began testing odor intensities and qualities as related to ingesting the test material. In addition he noted changes in mood. There were several surprises. Using four test vials, 10, 25, 50, and 100 milligrams of thiamine, a test panel of twenty research subjects fell into two clearly defined groups.

Group One reported that the odors increased in intensity from "just noticeable" at 10 milligrams, getting a little stronger at 25 and 50 milligrams, while becoming medium in strength at 100 milligrams. The qualitative changes—what the tablets smelled like and whether the odor was pleasant or unpleasant—changed from "no quality detectable" at 10 milligrams to "very sweet and pleasant" at 100 milligrams. This group also reported a definite change in mood, from "feeling low," "bored," and "dull," to feeling stimulated emotionally and "being definitely more alert mentally."

Group Two respondents reported changes in the opposite direction: intensity and odor quality at 10 milligrams was "strong, sharp, and unpleasant," while at 100 milligrams no odor could be detected, but they reported a "gassy" or "nose prickling" sensation. Mood changes ranged from "feeling good" at the beginning of the test to "feeling depressed," "irritable," and "generally down" emotionally and mentally at 100 milligrams.

This fascinating bit of research was the beginning of the development of what Watson calls "Psychochemical Types," which he has described and explained in *Nutrition and Your Mind.*

He spent all of his research time between 1948 and 1954, while teaching at the University of Southern California, on the problem of separating the vitamins, minerals, and trace elements into the Group I or Group II pattern of odor responses—depending on whether they pushed the oxidation rate up or down.

The scale of the research broadened in 1955, when Watson began working at the W. C. Kalash Laboratories. The laboratories provided not only laboratory tests on patients, medical examinations, and nutritional supplements for patients, but also a medical consultant, and later, a biochemist who specialized in mineral metabolism.

By 1961 Watson had developed vitamin-mineral formulas for both Type I and Type II patients (slow and fast oxidizers). He had also been able to isolate blood variables which would indicate which Psychochemical Type a given patient might be. In addition, the project had achieved a remarkable recovery rate for seriously disturbed mentally ill patients by using the appropriate vitamin-mineral formulas, plus the nutritional program best suited to the patient's type.

In 1961 Watson and several colleagues created the Lancaster Foundation for Scientific Research in Pasadena.

His first activity there was to collect, organize, and analyze statistically the data he had obtained in his six years at the Kalash Laboratories. He submitted the resulting paper to *Psychological Reports,* who not only accepted, but published the article as a separate, bound monograph. Its title was *Differences in Intermediary Metabolism in Mental Illness.* This work appears as an appendix in *Nutrition and Your Mind,* and is the scientific basis for the book.

Watson had been using the odor test, collecting patients' responses ever since 1948 when he was a professor at the University of Southern California. He spent at least half of his time between 1954 and 1961 trying to penetrate the jungle of odor responses and relate them to blood and psychological test scores. The range and variety of responses to single test samples such as Vitamin B_1 was simply staggering. There were thousands of odor protocols on each test substance, but there seemed to be no patterns of response among patients who had identical blood-test profiles.

Watson had established a rough, many-valued pattern that he personally—with his twenty years' experience—could interpret with high validity (over 90 percent) which correlated with blood tests and patients' improvement. The problem was how to standardize the test so that others could use it.

Eventually Watson hit on the idea of a *forced*-choice test, weighing the responses to a group of six substances numerically and correlating these numbers with blood test and psychological test scores.

He acquired a computer capable of factor analysis and spent the next year analyzing the data to discover "odor contexts" and constructed a standardized test. At Lancaster, he was able to numerically weigh the patients' responses and compare their scores with both blood and psychological tests, and with degrees of improvements in their illnesses.

The results were astonishing. The odor test scores correlated positively with the blood and psychological test scores, and with the patients' improvement. Frequently the blood tests would yield inconclusive results, leaving Watson in a trial and error situation in classifying the patient and selecting the best treatment.

The odor test *eliminated* this most vexing problem: it *always* yielded a score which could be translated into a treatment strategy.

He made up a dozen odor kits, and sent them out to psychiatrists and psychologists who were using *Nutrition and Your Mind* as a basis for treatment. The results were highly successful—one therapist who has been using psychochemical treatment for about ten years found the odor test the single most reliable instrument he possessed for classifying patients and determining their progress through the recovery period.

The Psychochemical Odor Test will be available in health food stores throughout the country under the Edom Laboratories label or you can make your own. The vitamin-mineral supplements for the various psychochemical types will also be available in health food stores under the Edom Laboratories label. If you have a serious difficulty in interpreting the results, even after consulting the text carefully, speak to a doctor. If the doctor is unable to resolve it, ask him or her to write to Dr. Watson in care of the publisher.

Index